MEDICAL PRACTICE MANAGEMENT

Body of Knowledge Review
Second Edition

VOLUME 4

Human Resource Management

Medical Group Management Association
102 Inverness Terrace East
Englewood, CO 80112-5306
877.275.6462
mgma.com

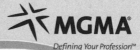

Medical Group Management Association® (MGMA®) publications are intended to provide current and accurate information and are designed to assist readers in becoming more familiar with the subject matter covered. Such publications are distributed with the understanding that MGMA does not render any legal, accounting, or other professional advice that may be construed as specifically applicable to an individual situation. No representations or warranties are made concerning the application of legal or other principles discussed by the authors to any specific factual situation, nor is any prediction made concerning how any particular judge, government official, or other person will interpret or apply such principles. Specific factual situations should be discussed with professional advisors.

PRODUCTION CREDITS
Publisher: Marilee E. Aust
Composition: Glacier Publishing Services, Inc.
Cover Design: Ian Serff, Serff Creative Group, Inc.

LIBRARY OF CONGRESS CATALOGING IN PUBLICATION DATA

Human resource management.
   p. ; cm. — (Medical practice management body of knowledge review
(2nd ed.) ; v. 4)
   Includes bibliographical references and index.
   ISBN 978-1-56829-333-2 (alk. paper)
1. Medical offices—Management. 2. Medicine—Practice. 3. Medical personnel.
4. Personnel Management. I. Medical Group Management Association. II. Series.
   [DNLM: 1. Practice Management, Medical—organization & administration.
2. Health Manpower—organization & administration. 3. Personnel Management—
methods. W 80 H918 2009]
   R728.H786 2009
   610.68—dc22

                                                                    2008044473

Printed in the United States of America
10 9 8 7 6 5 4 3 2 1

Dedication

To our colleagues in the profession
of medical practice management
and to the groups that support us
in our efforts to serve our profession.

Body of Knowledge Review Series — Second Edition

Contents

Preface

HUMAN RESOURCE MANAGEMENT, formerly known as personnel management, is part of every medical practice executive's responsibilities. Although small medical practices generally do not have a human resource department, as a practice grows in complexity and size, it often develops a function or department to provide human resource management. Human resource management is committed to making sure that the right number of people with the appropriate skills are in place to accomplish the medical practice's goals and objectives.

Maintaining an efficient and effective human resource function is one of the most important tasks of a medical practice executive. The medical practice has to care for its staff and attract and retain the best employees. The human resource function of managing employees and addressing their needs and wants is a constant challenge. However, a function that exclusively focuses on the employees without an organizational commitment to increase patient satisfaction through a cultural change will ultimately fall short on improving service. A well-run medical practice with a strong vision, mission, goals, and objectives will use its human resource function to develop, implement, and maintain excellent programs in salary and wage administration, benefits administration, procedures and policies, recruitment, appraisal and evaluation, employee relations, training and development, and reward and recognition. The key to that success will be grounded in excellent service and quality patient care.

Human resources must therefore focus its commitment to a service culture that brings physicians and employees together to improve patient, physician, and employee satisfaction. A commitment focused on service to people (patients, employees, physicians) fosters a transformation to service excellence. The medical practice that focuses its effort on excellent service will differentiate itself from the competition. The human resource function can help facilitate the accountability of that service from physicians, administrators, and staff. The shared commitment and cooperation of these groups is critical for a culture of service to evolve meaningfully and to make a difference.

The purpose of this volume is to offer a set of resources to promote ideas regarding the human resource function and to help the medical practice executive better understand the elements and components of human resources.

Body of Knowledge Review Series Contributors

Geraldine Amori, PhD, ARM, CPHRM
Douglas G. Anderson, FACMPE
James A. Barnes, MBA
Fred Beck, JD
Jerry D. Callahan Jr., CPA
Anthony J. DiPiazza, CPA
David N. Gans, MSHA, FACMPE
Robert L. Garrie, MPA, RHIA
Edward Gulko, MBA, FACMPE, FACHE, LNHA
Kenneth T. Hertz, CMPE
Steven M. Hudson, CFP, CFS, CRPC
Jerry Lagle, MBA, CPA, FACMPE
Michael Landers
Gary Lewins, FACMPE, CPA, FHFMA
Ken Mace, MA, CMPE
Jeffrey Milburn, MBA, CMPE
Michael A. O'Connell, MHA, FACMPE, CHE
Dawn M. Oetjen, PhD, MHA
Reid M. Oetjen, PhD, MSHSA
Pamela E. Paustian, MSM, RHIA
David Peterson, MBA, FACMPE
Lisa H. Schneck, MSJ
Frederic R. Simmons Jr., CPA
Thomas E. Sisson, CPA
Donna J. Slovensky, PhD, RHIA, FAHIMA
Jerry M. Trimm, PhD, FHIMSS
Stephen L. Wagner, PhD, FACMPE
Lee Ann H. Webster, MA, CPA, FACMPE
Susan Wendling-Aloi, MPA, FACMPE
Warren C. White Jr., FACMPE
Lawrence Wolper, MBA, FACMPE, CMC
Lorraine C. Woods, FACMPE
James R. Wurts, FACMPE

Learning Objectives

AFTER READING THIS VOLUME, the medical practice executive will be able to accomplish the following tasks:

- Coordinate the recruitment and orientation process of clinical and nonclinical staff;

- Manage the retention of clinical and nonclinical staff;

- Develop and monitor an effective staffing strategy;

- Develop and implement staff compensation and benefit plans;

- Provide systems, processes, and structure for administrative and clinical training for medical providers, employees, and students;

- Establish systems and processes for awareness, education, and compliance with employment laws and regulatory standards; and

- Provide personal commitment to enhance knowledge, skills, and abilities in health care administration.

**The Ties
That Bind**[1]

Now that you've found that ideal physician, how do you keep him or her? Physician recruitment is only half of the equation of a successful recruitment effort for a medical practice. Retention is the other half.

In an online survey, LocumTenens.com found that 84 percent of responding physicians considered a physician retention plan "very important" or "important" to their level of satisfaction, yet only 10 percent stated that their organizations employed any kind of physician retention initiative.[2]

So is anyone responding to this indicator?

■ Retain Physicians as Patient Demand Surges

A confluence of factors demonstrates medical organizations' recognition of the importance of retaining physicians. While numerical projections vary, there is general agreement that by the year 2020 we will see a significant physician shortage. This will occur in tandem with a wave of "baby boomers" reaching Medicare age in 2011 and spanning at least 10 years. More patients, fewer providers equal more work volume.

Physician morale appears to be on the decline. Practices confront shrinking reimbursement and increasing regulatory and bureaucratic pressures. The financial squeeze pushes providers to see more patients. The Internet has empowered patients with a wealth of information – empower-ment that may result in loss of respect for providers.[3]

Physicians see retention initiatives as important. Their morale is dropping, their ranks are thinning. The cost to replace them is high: One estimate puts the price to replace a physician in a primary care practice at $250,000.[4]

■ Developing an Effective Physician Retention Program

An effective physician retention program begins prior to the recruitment process, works through that process, and continues through the new recruit's tenure with the practice. It involves the physician's family as well. It considers work-life balance. It factors in the physician's practice issues and the needs of the community. It is, at its core, a program that recognizes the importance of the physician-practice relationship and the many dimensions that affect its stability.

It's a good idea to have written plans for both physician recruit-ment and retention. This ensures consistency and allows a thorough evaluation of strategies and tactics. In addition to recruitment and retention plans, practices often develop a physician compact or a physician policy manual.

The compact is generally a one- or two-page document outlin-ing what the practice expects of new physicians and what physi-cians may expect from the practice. The compact is typically written on a macro level, staying above practice operations, policies, and procedures.

The policy manual provides nitty-gritty detail. It addresses spe-cific issues such as call coverage, patient transfer, continuing med-ical education, and time off.

For either document to have traction in the group, it must be developed with the input and participation of the providers.

◼ Recruitment

Before you attempt to hire and keep physicians, you must understand the nature of your organization: its practice style, culture, age distribution of physicians, formal and informal network dynamics, governance, and leadership style.

Determine the personality type of a physician who would make a good fit with your practice and your community. If you engage a recruiter to assist you in the search, develop specific, well-articulated criteria for candidate selection. Clinical skills and competence are musts, but given the rate of turnover, the costs of replacing a physician and increased pressure on providers, it's critical that you perform as much preselection as possible before on-site interviews.

For example, a cardiology group entertained a candidate for a site visit and learned that his spouse wanted to be located near her family. She was disinclined to even consider an offer from this group – about 12 states away. If practice leaders had established their job-candidate criteria at the outset of the recruitment effort – including an individual's strong interest in their area – this site visit could have been avoided, saving time and money for all involved.

Clearly articulate the practice's vision, mission, and values. If your organization doesn't already have these outlined, do it now. Candidates – and existing physicians and staff – will want to know where the practice stands and where leaders see it going. Discuss the mission, vision, and values when screening candidate physicians – prior to the on-site interview – to ensure congruity. Be clear about the group's expectations of physicians, and of physicians' expectations of the group.

The physician's spouse and family are also critical to candidate retention. Physicians leave employment situations because of a poor cultural fit, lack of an adequate support network for the spouse and children, or poor fit with the community.[5] It is vital to identify the spouse's needs and interests during the selection and before the site-visit process. Once the candidate (and perhaps the spouse) is sitting in front of you, address those needs and interests. (See Exhibit 1.)

EXHIBIT 1
Get a Cultural Fit[6]

A key to retention is hiring doctors who fit your practice's culture. To determine this, ask certain questions. Have physicians describe situations when they had to:

- Adapt to changes they didn't support;
- Deal with a miscommunication with a patient or employee;
- Handle a situation without direction from a supervisor; and
- Deal with someone who didn't perform up to expectations.

Their answers reveal how they react to everyday situations and whether they're a cultural fit.

Employment

If you did your homework in recruiting, there's a good chance you drew a competent physician candidate who fits the practice style and culture, and whose personal vision and mission match those of the organization. The new associate and his family will fit nicely into the community.

Now, ensure that you have an organized retention effort to guarantee that your new associate has a positive and rewarding experience.

Too often, new physicians receive little or no mentoring; they're just thrown into the practice. Mentoring newcomers can pay big dividends in an associate's comfort level with his or her new job and regard for the organization. Identify a senior member of the practice to serve as a mentor to the new doctor on patient care issues, and who can guide him or her through the potential minefield of a new practice situation.

It is also important that the practice establish a formal feedback mechanism to ensure that the new associate understands how he or she is doing. Be sure this communication is physician to physician – the administrator does not need to be in the middle of this discussion.

◼ Retention Strategies Promote Openness, Information-Sharing

Transparency within the medical practice helps foster the development of future leaders. Consider including new associates in meetings with the partners. While they don't necessarily have a vote, the younger physicians benefit from involvement in discussions. They observe the governance and decision-making style of the practice and feel respected by the senior members.

Likewise, share financial and productivity information with new associates. Secrecy does not build an environment of trust and does not promote physician retention. Develop standard reports and a time to meet with the new associates. Let them know what is happening. Make them a part of the practice early on and you will receive loyalty down the road.

Information-sharing is vital in a physician retention program. So, too, is the management of expectations. Discussing physician compact items – the give and get – establishes a clear set of expectations for both the practice and the new associate. Regularly monitor those expectations to ensure they are being met, and if not, remedy the situation earlier rather than later.

Consider using questionnaires and interviews with new physicians to bring issues to light. Questions might include:

- What is your personal mission?
- Why did you join this group?
- Have your expectations been met? If not, why?
- What are the top three issues you believe the group faces in the next year?

- Describe your involvement in decision making.
- Describe your level of clinical satisfaction.

The responses can reveal both individual and group issues needing attention.

◪ Physician Retention Helps a Practice Succeed

The confluence of an increasing patient load, a decreasing number of providers, declining reimbursement, and increasing costs create a situation in which it is increasingly important to retain the physicians you recruit.

Success requires clarity of purpose, vision on the part of the practice, and a thorough and thoughtful screening and interview process. Once the candidate becomes a new associate in your group, transparency, communication, support, and mentoring will work to protect your investment for a long time.

Current Human Resource Management Issues

THE HUMAN RESOURCES PROFESSION is at a crossroads and needs to face up to its challenges or become a marginal contributor to organizational success. The medical practice executive is expected to substantially change the mix of activities in human resources to contribute to organizational strategy and effectiveness. The practice executive is challenged, however, with the wide mix of issues in the Human Resource Management domain.

Medical practices are constantly faced with issues to cut costs as managed care companies and government insurers reduce reimbursement and external groups (e.g., malpractice insurers, vendors) increase costs for services provided. Cost-cutting measures typically fall between reducing staff wages and benefits or improving efficiencies in systems and processes so additional staff don't need to be hired. The Human Resource Management domain focuses on recruiting qualified people, providing competitive wages and benefits, training and educating, team building, managing performance, maintaining a positive work environment, supporting legal business practices and worker conditions, and carrying out the best human resources (HR) strategy for the future.

Some of the expected HR trends and their resultant challenges in the market include:

- Technical and professional employee needs are increasing as work becomes more technology oriented, and nontechnical employee jobs are also being impacted by technological advances. As "Baby Boomers" (those born between 1946 and 1964) continue to retire in the near future, the unavailability of skilled workers will intensify. A consequence is that the professional concerned with human resources will need to come up with creative ways to recruit qualified people and will need to be more proactive with succession planning.

- The training of nontechnical employees will shift to employers in the form of on-the-job training, as lower educational standards produce graduates unprepared for work. (Employers may even have to help with such basic skills as reading, writing, and arithmetic.)

- The lack of loyalty shown by both the employer and employee is changing the work culture. The labor force will be more transient, and staff members are likely to leave one job for another for a slight increase in pay. In addition, the employer's bottom-line approach will lead to more layoffs than ever before. The HR professional will therefore need to be more flexible and creative in work-force needs.

- Medical practices will have a greater demand to be customer focused and require that employees have service and teamwork skills and be empowered to solve problems quickly.

- HR professionals will need a work force with strong "soft" skills, such as a positive attitude, motivation, adaptability, and energy; and will be challenged to develop selection methods that evaluate these criteria. The HR focus will be on the whole employee, including training, counseling, and coaching.

- Outsourcing of staff and services will continue to be considered and will create conflicts with labor unions and loyal employees who see this strategy as a threat to future jobs.

- As performance and outcomes become the "bottom line," HR professionals will need to develop effective performance management systems.

- As resources become scarce, new models for employment will need to be developed with the public and private sector, including job sharing, loaned employees, outsourced employees, and other collaborative models.

- Labor unions' traditional practices are becoming outdated in today's market and have resulted in a decline in union memberships. Unions will require new approaches with management to address more beneficial solutions.

The executive concerned with human resources in the future will not only focus on payroll and benefit administration, but will provide opportunities to employees to customize service, including skill-building training, personalized coaching, resources for more effective problem solving, and better and simpler ways to track information. A clear understanding and knowledge of the Human Resource Management domain by the medical practice executive is needed to ensure the success of the medical practice.

Knowledge Needs

THE KNOWLEDGE BASE required to perform human resource management functions is comprehensive, incorporating the fields of finance, law, management, and information technology. This domain's published literature is as varied as it is complex, from rightsizing the medical practice to preparing manuals on job descriptions and personnel policies. Some of the literature is unique to medical practices, whereas other literature draws from the plethora of resources in manufacturing and the service industry. The need for advice and help in the Human Resource Management domain continues to grow as practice executives confront issues unique to them in the 21st century and seek answers to their complex problems.

The medical practice executive should perform both simple and complex management skills to promote employee productivity and organizational performance. The medical practice executive should:

- Understand federal and state employment laws by accurately recording and reporting compliance with regulations;

- Have knowledge of compensation and benefits administration to manage a program that best meets practice needs;

- Collect and analyze data on personnel issues and resolve the identified matters;

- Maintain currency on human resources (HR) issues pertaining to employment, staffing, compensation, and regulations;

- Educate staff on best HR practices, including employee development, training, education, and communication;

- Advise management on personnel issues, including disciplinary action, labor disputes, employee morale, and consistent administration of personnel policies; and

- Use appropriate management information system software to gather, analyze, and present HR data.

Demonstrating mastery of the Human Resource Management domain outlined within the *Medical Practice Management Body of Knowledge, second edition,* requires the medical practice executive to understand the balance between management and employees and to make sure that all needs are met in the areas of administration, recruitment, compensation and benefits, training and development, health and safety, and employee relations. Formal education in human resources can lead to an associate's, bachelor's, master's, or doctoral degree. Course work includes instruction in personnel and organization policy, labor relations, labor law and regulations, motivation and compensation, career management, employee testing and assessment, recruitment and selection, employee- and job-training programs, and management of human resources programs and operations, among others. In addition, special certifications offered through the Society for Human Resource Management validate a person's knowledge in a particular human resources area. The medical practice executive may choose to pursue a self-directed course of study in human resources instead of seeking a formal degree or certification.

Many medical practice executives have staff that perform the human resource function and will therefore need to provide executive oversight and direction rather than directly running the functions. Choosing the right people for these leadership roles is critical and requires the medical practice executive to have a thorough understanding of the Human Resource Management domain. The executive needs to ensure that the HR department accurately represents and promotes the vision and values of the organization through its practices, and that it is approachable and credible and seen as a resource for all employees. The medical practice executive therefore has the responsibility for a successfully run HR department, primarily to:

- Develop HR policies and programs for the organization;
- Recommend employee relations practices to establish positive relationships;
- Address legal requirements and regulations;
- Establish wage and salary structures; pay policies; and performance, benefit, and safety and health programs;
- Establish recruitment and placement practices; and
- Develop training programs.

A medical practice executive who is knowledgeable in the Human Resource Management domain through mastery of essential skills allows for a positive environment of increased participation, higher morale, enhanced employee engagement, and improved team performance. Human resource management serves both a supportive function and one of leading strategy and effective change. The medical practice executive learns the Human Resource Management domain and its necessary skills and knowledge through formal education, self-directed learning, and experience in the field, all combining to achieve competence in the domain. Although exclusive self-directed learning can be pursued to master the domain, experience helps to solidify the knowledge, along with educational programs and workshops.

Chapter 1   **Recruiting Staff**

■ Recruiting from Inside the Organization

A medical practice that posts all positions internally prior to posting them externally has a "promotion-from-within" philosophy. This approach conveys to the work force that it values hiring from within prior to considering external candidates. Usually a position is posted internally for several days and those candidates are interviewed prior to external candidates being considered. Some medical practices will post the position internally, concurrently post the position for the external marketplace, and hire the best-qualified candidate.

Sometimes an internal referral is the best way to find a new staff person. An employee will usually refer someone who is thought to be a good worker because referring an unproductive worker will reflect poorly on that employee.

■ Recruiting External Candidates

Advertising Strategy

There are limited dollars to advertise job openings. The medical practice executive determines how that money will be allocated. Newspaper ads in local and regional papers, television commercials, Internet banners, magazine ads in professional journals, and direct mail are all examples of advertising strategies that medical practices have used to recruit new staff.

Temporary Agencies

Temporary agencies can provide staff needed for a time-specific project or activity. They can also be resources for permanent employees. Hiring temporary agency staff allows a medical practice executive to determine whether a person possesses the necessary skills to perform the job on a continual basis and could fit within the organizational culture. Usually, if a company wants to hire a temporary agency worker, the agency charges a placement fee, which could be as much as 100 percent of the employee's first year's salary.

Internet Job-Posting Services

With the growth of the Internet, jobs can now be advertised on the medical practice's Website. An Internet search for a specific job or organization will bring up the job posting. This type of resource simplifies the job search for prospective candidates.

Search Firms

A search firm is a professional service provided to a medical practice to attract, hire, and develop staff who will hold jobs that are key to achieving the medical practice's goals and objectives. The service is paid by the medical practice, not the hired person. Possible job candidates are presented to the medical group by the search firm based on employer-specified requirements. The use of a search firm is meant to save the medical practice executive's time and money because identifying, qualifying, and reviewing potential candidates can be an expensive effort requiring tremendous effort.

When a search firm is hired on a contingency basis, that firm will earn a fee only if a job candidate is hired and retained by the medical practice. A *headhunter* is a common term used for a contingent firm because the majority of the firm's effort is based on getting the potential candidate in front of the medical practice.

In contrast, hiring a retained search firm means that the medical practice has a signed contract with the firm to hire a candidate, and these two groups work exclusively with each other to find that person. Also, the search firm is paid in advance, in whole or in part, prior to the candidate being hired.

Regardless of the type of search firm contacted, the medical group and firm must correctly fit the potential job candidate with the skills needed for the job to achieve a satisfactory hiring outcome.

Community Placement Services

A community placement service helps to link prospective job candidates to interested employers. These services may focus on working with students, new graduates, or displaced workers. The placement service is able to help the prospective job candidate develop a skill base, enhance the candidate's resume, help him or her gain a better understanding of various job opportunities within the community, and develop networks and support systems of people who can provide letters of recommendation, references, and possible job options.

■ Selection

Human resources must be fair and consistent in its hiring practices. A person who starts working in the medical practice without following any of the procedures or policies may engender a complaint being filed by other co-workers. Common mistakes are failing to post a position internally, failing to complete an employment application, or a person starting to work without having completed a drug screen or health physical. Even if the need to fill a position is urgent, it should never be done at the expense of following the process accepted by the medical practice. It is critical that the medical practice executive follow all legal practices and comply with all rules and regulations toward fair hiring practices.

There is a basic process for employee selection and customized applications, depending on the position:

- *Employment application form.* The application is the same regardless of the position. An application should be completed prior to conducting any interviews. The application will ask for information such as demographics, education, work history, references, and criminal record. The employee will sign the application, indicating that the information is correct and authorizing a release to the medical practice to verify the information.

- *Equal employment opportunity (EEO) factors (e.g., advertising, recruiting, record-keeping).* Careful records should be kept for any position being recruited. If a person later files a complaint against the medical practice due to violation of EEO factors, the practice would want to demonstrate that its process was fair and consistent, and complied with the law.

- *Interviewing (screening, behavior-based).* Screening interviews may be held on the telephone to determine the candidate's level of interest and skills for the position. Behavior-based interviews present the candidate with scenarios and ask how he or she would respond to those situations.

- *Panel interviews.* A panel interview may be a peer interview by people with whom the candidate potentially would work. This approach builds consensus from co-workers and allows them input into the process.

- *Open-ended questions.* Open-ended questions require more than just a "yes" or "no" answer. They encourage the candidate to discuss issues and share information about his or her background, experience, skills, and abilities, so that the employer can determine whether the candidate will be a good fit for the position.

- *Testing (written, performance).* Some positions require a written or performance test to demonstrate competency in a job requirement. A medical secretary who is required to type 40 words a minute would take a typing test, or a file clerk would take a test showing the ability to file alphabetically and numerically.

- *Reference checks.* A job candidate consenting to reference checks allows the employer to talk to other people about the candidate and ask questions without fear of being sued or risking legal action. Some previous employers will give out only limited information, including the employee's position title, starting and ending dates of employment, and rate of pay. Others will answer questions about a past employee's quality and quantity of work, time and attendance, customer service background, and whether the employer would rehire the employee.

- *Criminal investigation and background checks.* Questions on the job application ask the potential employee if he or she has ever been convicted of a misdemeanor or felony. An official background check is usually conducted after an employment offer and prior to the employee's first day of work to verify that the employee doesn't have any undisclosed criminal history.

- *Offer of employment.* An offer of employment is usually made to the candidate with some time specified before a response is needed. If the position is accepted, a written confirmation is sent to the candidate confirming title, rate of pay, contingencies of employment, and start date.

- *Health information and physical exams.* An employment offer may be contingent on the person providing health information and passing a physical exam. There may be a pre-employment drug physical to verify that the person is drug-free. Failure to pass any of these tests may result in the employment offer being withdrawn.

Chapter 2 **Orienting, Retaining, and Disciplining Staff**

▨ The Link Between Physician Retention and Orientation[7]

When developing and implementing a formal physician orientation program, link the objectives of physician retention and orientation. An orientation program permits newly hired physicians to meet senior management and learn about the practice's strategies, market, managed care relationships, clinical programs, residency teaching, rotations, continuing education, research opportunities, risk management, and recruiting – to name a few.[8]

Linking your physician orientation and retention programs begins with the components listed in Exhibit 2.

When the employment market was more fluid, practices regarded retention-related orientation programs as an afterthought of the recruitment function. As a result, physician orientation was often limited to a rote explanation of the rules, compensation, and other company policies necessary to ensure smooth personnel functions. But now the emphasis in orientation is moving from the end of the recruitment function to the beginning of the retention process.

EXHIBIT 2

Linking Physician Orientation and Retention Programs[9]

Establish board policy	Put the elements of this plan, including goals and objectives, into writing and get approval at the board level.
Designate responsibility	Specific individuals should monitor, manage, and be held responsible for retention duties; larger practices should consider establishing a retention committee.
Recruit wisely	Many issues that lead physicians to leave a practice can be discovered through careful screening, assessment, and interviewing of potential recruits.
Conduct thorough orientation	Plan to show newcomers the community, including hospitals, clinic sites, and nursing home with which the practice interacts.
Introduce newcomers	Introduce newcomers to other physicians in the community, including those they will deal with for referrals or consultations, and certain other key players from outside the practice, such as administrators of referring facilities.
Develop a marketing plan	Show newcomers how the medical practice will make them known to the community.
Implement a mentor system	Don't choose a mentor who is a superior or subordinate to the physician.
Implement a mentor system for the physician's spouse	Finding someone of the spouse's gender to help him/her adapt to the community is especially important when the physician has relocated.
Integrate into the community	Help the physician and family integrate into the community. Some communities, especially small ones, can be hard to break into, so take extra steps if needed.
Give positive reinforcement	Figure out informal ways to give the newcomer a "pat on the back."
Conduct exit interviews	Interview all physicians who leave. Departing members of the practice can be frank and reveal issues that create difficulty for newcomers.

Managing Expectations

Managing expectations is one of the keys to successful retention. To do so involves fostering two-way communication, implementing a physician recognition program, and providing forums to review opportunities.

Physician supervisors should schedule regular individual and group meetings with new doctors to answer questions, discuss concerns, and provide feedback. Make resolution of questions, concerns, and complaints a priority to keep morale high.

Holding regional or systemwide forums twice a year is a good way to meet with the group and encourage two-way communication. Smaller practices should get all physicians and nonphysician providers together to discuss issues.

Practices and physicians must develop and maintain common expectations of the group's mission, values, and goals to work effectively as a team. In simpler times, this understanding could be unwritten. But given today's pressures and complexities, it's a good idea to write down the group's common mission, values, and expectations. Review them periodically. The factors of successful groups include:

- A written statement of mission and values;
- Measurable quality and business goals;
- Measurement and review of the practice's progress; and
- Agreed-upon expectations among physicians.[10]

Integrating the Culture

A physician orientation program that embodies practice culture can assist physician retention by accelerating the integration process for new hires.

In a nutshell, culture is the "way we do things." It is a system of shared beliefs, values, and behaviors within an organization.

Indicators that a practice exhibits cultural integration include physicians who are:

- Willing to delegate authority and give up individual autonomy;

- Able to work collaboratively to solve problems;

- Committed and/or willing to follow group goals and directives;

- Accepting of consolidation of practices and economies of scale;

- Willing to share income, expense, and/or governance;

- Focused on the long term and the short term; and

- Willing to deal with problems of other group physicians.[11]

Cultural integration should also include communicating the governance structure. Typically, a practice elects a small-sized board or executive committee, with clear differentiation between the roles of the board (policy making) and management (policy implementation).

Finally, strong leadership – both physician and administrative – must exist for a successful cultural integration. The new physician(s) must be given appropriate accountabilities to ensure that they understand their roles and responsibilities.[12]

◼ Retaining and Developing Employees[13]

The performance management process – which includes performance planning, evaluation, and rating – is a vital aspect of human resource management. It is perhaps the most important and sometimes most troublesome aspect of the employer–employee relationship.

The results of the performance management process are used in setting individual goals and objectives; awarding salary increases; identifying promotional, transfer, and training opportunities; and determining potential disciplinary and termination actions. Often this aspect of management is the most vulnerable point of the employment relationship, generating the most complaints about management functions. These complaints occur because many performance evaluation systems are subjective and result in discriminatory management decisions based on arbitrary judgments. Vague and ill-defined performance criteria lend themselves to biased judgments and evaluations – and to litigation. Therefore, it is critical that employers have a performance management system that (1) accurately measures and improves employee performance, and (2) is legally defensible.

The impetus for developing an effective performance management process is very clear. Salaries and wages compose as much as 60 to 70 percent of a health care organization's total operating costs. There is a clear link between the successful organizational operation and the effective and efficient performance of its employees. A comprehensive performance management process can help the organization attract and retain highly qualified employees and ensure quality, cost-effective service. The result is the achievement of both employee and employer goals.

As patient expectations and demands increase, the quality of performance, whether of a physician, nurse, or other staff member, must also increase. Total quality performance management becomes more vital. To maintain and expand the current patient and financial base, medical practices need a performance management process that is contemporary and easy to administer – and that works.

Managers often have misguided and even counterproductive beliefs about why organizations have performance evaluation systems in the first place. Many of these beliefs occur because managers have poorly designed performance evaluation systems that focus on judging the employee as a person, rather than on evaluating the employee's job performance and behavior. As a result, performance interviews often reflect a parent–child relationship – an awkward situation that causes tension and distress for both the employee and the supervisor.

Many times, organizations poorly define the job criteria that will result in high levels of performance. They fail to encourage an employee's self-evaluation. They tie the performance process to administrative issues, such as compensation, rather than to development of the employee, the supervisor, and the organization.

Consider the word "performance" in performance management. This is what management is all about; that is, supervisors plan, organize, lead, and control performance. An effective performance management process enhances each of those tasks and results in improved productivity. Supervisors are expected to have insight into what goals to set, how to achieve those goals, how to organize work efforts appropriately, how to lead workers in the right direction, and how to monitor and control performance so that it stays on target.

An effective performance management process encompasses six components. These are:

1. Organizational goals and objectives;

2. Individual's performance and planning;

3. Employee performance measurements;

4. Performance reviews;

5. Ongoing feedback and coaching; and

6. Recognition and rewards.

The medical group should emphasize performance expectations up front, reinforce them consistently, and reward results regularly. Your group should provide a uniform and general framework for performance management that ensures employees know what is expected of them and supervisors know how to establish a job-related basis for planning, managing, and evaluating performance.

Performance Planning and Evaluation Overview

Although state and federal statutes do not mandate performance evaluations for private employees, an employer generally cannot be held liable for failing to give an employee a performance assessment. There are exceptions to these rules. If an employer makes a promise to an employee that s/he will receive an evaluation, and the employee does not get an evaluation, the employer could, in theory, be found liable under a breach of contract. In this situation, the employer made a promise to the employee, either oral or written. The employee relied on the promise, the employer broke the promise, and the employee was harmed.

Most often, promises of performance evaluations are written either in an employment offer letter, an employee contract, or the employee handbook. If the employee handbook states that "employees will receive annual performance evaluations," that statement can create an enforceable right to a performance evaluation. On the other hand, a slight wording change can have important legal ramifications. If the employee handbook states that "employees should receive annual performance evaluations," a court is much more likely to rule that an annual performance review is not a "right" of the employee, but rather a "goal" of the employer.

You should review employment offer letters, employee contracts, and employee handbooks to eliminate language that may obligate the group to give performance evaluations.

There are several pitfalls that the medical group's managers and supervisors can avoid to protect the group from legal issues regarding performance. These are as follows:

Management Pitfalls

- Not developing and maintaining a sound performance process

- Not providing training about the process

- Not enforcing the use of the process

- Not ensuring appropriate uses of the process and relevant policies and procedures

- Not requiring legal advice before discharging an employee

- Not creating an employee performance evaluation appeal process

Supervisory Pitfalls

- Paying little attention to performance planning

- Giving inadequate feedback to employees

- Failing to observe and correct performance problems immediately

- Spending little time completing the required performance evaluation forms

- Neglecting to complete regular evaluations

- Not being honest and thorough

- Giving inflated ratings or favoring certain employees

- Not taking performance management seriously

Performance Evaluation Tools

There are many performance planning and evaluation tools; the paragraphs that follow describe some of these evaluation tools. Each has its advantages and disadvantages.

Critical Incident Rating

This approach is based on an appraiser's written observation of an employee's performance throughout a designated time period. The supervisor maintains a log to record an employee's performance during work incidents that are considered critical, such as dealing with a patient. These critical incidents are sometimes called significant occurrences. This performance log should contain examples of both satisfactory and unsatisfactory performance.

Because the critical incident report is similar to the essay, it relies heavily on the supervisor's verbal skills. Although it has the advantage of being job related, it can be biased by the incidents the supervisor chooses to record. It is a common mistake to record only incidents that the supervisor finds unsatisfactory. Supervisors forget to record incidents of exceptional performance because, in reality, they expect that type of behavior.

If done correctly, this approach is very time-consuming for the supervisor, requiring constant note taking and close observation. Employees consider such constant observation as micromanagement. Employees dislike having someone looking over their shoulders all day.

One positive use of this approach is to amplify specific job-related examples when using other formats. The approach is most useful, however, when dealing with performance problems. Documentation of critical incidents is a vital step in developing a performance improvement plan or preparing to discipline or terminate an employee.

Peer Review

The peer review method was originally designed for rating professional employees. It is frequently used in medical practices by and for physicians. In this process, a panel of colleagues confidentially rates each physician's performance. One of the main benefits of this system is that it allows for a credible rating by equals of a highly sophisticated work force.

Many health care organizations are redesigning peer/co-worker reviews so they can be used by any work group to evaluate employees in terms of performance factors such as patient relations, teamwork, and quality. In time, co-worker reviews may become an integral part of the total performance plan and evaluation process. The medical group will base these reviews on its own defined performance factors and standards.

There are several performance evaluation tools that require the evaluator to compare employees. These include:

- Paired comparison ranking, which involves comparing each employee in a job to all other employees in the group;

- Alternation ranking, which involves evaluating all workers in a job group against a standard measure; and

- Forced distribution ranking, which involves ranking employees on a universal measure according to a fixed proportion of the entire group.

One disadvantage of the ranking approach is that it focuses on the group rather than on the individual. It does not recognize that each person has a different level of experience in the job, has different strengths and weaknesses, and may be on a different development path. Most important, ranking fails to identify individual differences in performance or inform the individual employee on how performance can be improved.

360-Degree Evaluation

The 360-degree evaluation is a very popular approach used by all types of business. This approach involves getting evaluations from a variety of people who interact with an employee. It usually includes supervisors, co-workers, and staff from different departments who interact with the employee on a regular basis, subordinates, customers, suppliers, and others. This type of evaluation also requires that the employee complete a self-evaluation using the same format that other evaluators use.

The purpose of the 360-degree review is to achieve more accurate results of overall performance. It can highlight areas of needed improvement that prevent other workers from performing their duties. Implementing 360-degree reviews is not difficult if your group already uses a form of peer reviews. These reviews can be done on paper or online through secured access in the group's intranet. Once all questionnaires have been distributed to specific parties, completed, and submitted, the direct supervisor or a human resources representative tallies the scores, develops a performance improvement plan, and discusses the results with the employee. The results are given to the direct supervisor for review with the employee.

Performance Standard

A performance standard method can be used successfully as both a planning and evaluation tool. It focuses on general job-related factors that are applicable among all employees or across specific groups. This method is useful in reinforcing the performance factors that are important to a medical practice.

Factor definitions should be stated in behavioral language – for example, "Patient relations: Display of respect, patience, helpfulness to patients, friendly manner, appropriate acknowledgment of patient feelings, ability to deal with clients in a nondefensive manner." Legally, it is unacceptable to use personality traits or attitudes as performance criteria. The focus must be on performance factors that are specific and critical to the job.

Once the medical practice has determined the factors it values, the tool can be used for all employees, including management. This format allows for tailoring to each job. The supervisors should add two to four performance standards and behavioral comments that directly related to each employee's job. All factors should be discussed and agreed upon by the supervisor and the employee.

Performance measurement standards should be expressed in specific, measurable terms (e.g., quantity, quality, time, and cost). In addition, they should be both realistic and challenging.

A simple rating scale can be used with a performance standard tool. The rating scale can be numerical (e.g., from 1 being "unacceptable" to 5 being "outstanding"). The preferred approach is to scale by four levels (e.g., does not meet standard, meets standard, above standard, and exceeds standard). The word *standard* reinforces the concept of a performance standard of success. It does not mean "average." Rather, it means "fully acceptable," "competent," "proficient," or "hitting the mark."

An odd number of points on the scale can cause a tendency to grade in the middle. That is why many performance management experts prefer a scale with four points of measurement.

Once the factors and standards have been finalized, the supervisor implements the tool for performance planning immediately. For example, a new employee would not only receive a copy of his or her job description, but also a copy of the performance plan. The supervisor would explain the expectations, with modifications made to fit the new employee's skill and experience level. With all employees, the supervisor and employee can use the tool to plan performance for the next period.

The performance standard approach takes little time to develop and use, and it does not require extensive verbal skills. However, a rating by itself does not inform employees of their deficiencies or motivate them to improve their performance. Therefore, if this method is used, supervisors should include a descriptive comment about each performance factor to clarify the rating at evaluation time. The group practice could select six to ten performance standards for each job and then have the supervisor add two to four performance standards that are job specific for each staff member.

This approach also requires the assignment of an "importance weight" to each factor – that is, each factor is assigned a numerical value that reflects its importance in overall job performance. For example, quality might be given a weight of 50 percent. It is important for employees to know how important each factor is or what counts most. Again, this should be discussed at the beginning of each performance period to ensure that the supervisor and employee agree on the priorities.

This method takes some upfront time to develop in that supervisors must specify significant performance factors, the related standards, and the relative weights. However, once the tool is developed, it is very easy to use. It is a common-sense approach that facilitates effective communication between the supervisor and employee.

Criterion-Based Method

The criterion-based approach is another recommended option. It features more specific descriptions of performance factors. It can be used both as a planning tool at the start of the year and as an evaluation tool.

The criterion approach focuses on clearly defined criteria and standards. A criterion is a specific area of job performance that is used to evaluate an employee's performance.

A performance standard in a criterion-based approach is represented by a series of performance levels. Each level correlates to a particular performance rating for the criterion. For example, a rate of return on investment that is 0 to 3 percent might be rated as "does not meet standard."

The performance standard in this tool is a measurement device that is very specific so that performance expectations are very clear. The measurements should relate to quantity, quality, timeliness, and financial parameters. It should be expressed in numerical or behavioral terms to ensure validity and reliability.

Goal Setting

A goal-setting system involves negotiation between the supervisor and employee to establish performance objectives. It is used at the beginning of a performance period, which might be the probationary/training period or a complete year. One widely used technique is management by objectives (MBO). This technique involves mutual goal setting between supervisors and employees. The employee aims to meet the agreed-upon goals within a determined time period.

The MBO approach usually involves:

- A job review and goal-setting agreement by the supervisor and employee;

- Development of performance standards by both;

- A reality check to ensure that the objectives are achievable (i.e., that resources are available and that the employee has control over the outcome); and

- Ongoing discussion throughout the time period concerning the employee's performance in regard to the established objectives.

The main strength of the MBO approach is that it focuses on the organization's goals and objectives. It is directly tied to the strategic plan, so the employee is very aware of how his or her performance will affect the organization's success. In addition, employee input is stressed in order to improve commitment and performance.

One major drawback to the MBO process is that it may not work well for all types of jobs. For example, it may be difficult to tie the performance of a medical records clerk to specific organizational objectives.

In addition, the MBO approach may concentrate too heavily on results, ignoring the methods required to achieve the objectives. That is, it may become a matter of "winning the war, but killing all the troops in the process." It also is a time-consuming process because the supervisor must invest considerable time negotiating with each employee.

Variations of the MBO approach – where job goals are less directly tied to specific organizational objectives – offer considerable merit to medical practices. A goal-setting format that works well is one focused on major accountabilities related to the job description. In this approach, three to six major accountabilities are identified. The supervisor and employee negotiate expected results in terms of objectives and measurable standards. These may be weighted to indicate priority.

Some medical practices use the same tool for all employees regardless of job function or exempt/nonexempt status. Others will identify key performance factors that are mandatory for every employee – for example, patient relations – and then add other performance factors for specific jobs or levels. Using separate forms for management and nonmanagement is strongly recommended. This is an effective way of reinforcing performance factors that pertain to management. Each group practice must decide on the management factors most important to them. These factors may include leadership, creativity, innovation, decision making, fiscal responsibility, and strategic planning.

Promotions

Employees often are an overlooked resource. Your medical group knows much more about its current staff's work history and potential than it does about new recruits. Often the expensive initial cost of recruiting, orienting, and training new employees can be saved by promoting competent employees – those who already have demonstrated their loyalty, stability, and work performance – to higher-level jobs.

The hope of a promotion to a better job and a chance to improve salary are very important to most employees, so a promotion-from-within policy can be an effective motivator. Employees will strive to do their best and often obtain additional training and/or education to increase their chances of being promoted.

A promotion-from-within policy increases employee morale, improves productivity and long-term employment, reduces turnover, and is cost-effective. Recruiting and training costs are significantly reduced when employees are promoted rather than hired from outside the group. Depending on the level of a vacant position, it can take six months to a year for a new employee to become fully productive. Current employees are already familiar with the medical group, its policies, and employees; they must only learn the new job.

A promotion-from-within policy also means that a promoted employee can do several jobs. Having employees who are able to perform many jobs makes for a more flexible work force. Such a policy means that lower-level jobs become available, which are usually easier to fill. Of course, your group needs to fill every position with the best qualified person, but your group should also try to build morale and increase productivity. Be aware, however, that in today's climate of downsizing, mergers, and integration, promotions may not be as available as in the past. Therefore, cross-training and job enhancement, in addition to promotions, have become a major focus.

Implementing a Promotion Program

The human resources (HR) specialist should coordinate your promotion program. Supervisors and managers usually will not oppose promotions, but they are often unaware of qualified employees who might be eligible for and interested in a promotion. To be effective and respected by employees, support for the promotion program must begin with top management.

Effective promotion program elements are:

- Job posting;
- Job bidding;
- Use of employee records;
- Skills inventory;
- Staff coordination;
- Good record-keeping; and
- Employee development programs.

These elements are crucial to recruiting present employees for job openings in your medical group. The typical procedure is to post job vacancies on online message boards, bulletin boards, or through e-mail, with a brief description of the job duties and qualifications.

Another procedure is job bidding, where interested employees complete an employee job bid form and submit it to the HR department before the closing deadline. The job bidding system should be open to all full- and part-time employees working at least 20 hours per week. In most cases, employees should be employed by the group for at least six consecutive months before being promoted.

An up-to-date skills inventory of your present staff is an effective method of locating internal employees eligible for promotion. Information on employees' skills, education, training, and interests can be pulled from an electronic database or employee records and evaluated.

Another critical element of the job promotion program is assigning someone to be responsible for coordinating the program. This person can counsel employees who are interested in transfers or promotional opportunities, or who are considering resigning to obtain a position outside your group.

Finally, an effective promotion program relies on good employee records. This helps your group practice report results to the Equal Employment Opportunity Commission, if necessary. Managers should also publicize efforts to promote employees. Your group should keep statistics on the number and kinds of employees who are either transferred or promoted during each year. Analyzing, reviewing, and reporting results contribute to the continued success of the program.

Well-motivated, productive, and efficient employees are a valuable commodity. Supervisors should urge outstanding employees to seek promotions. Your medical group should encourage its supervisors and managers to endorse your promotion program and refrain from blocking transfers and promotions of qualified employees. A supervisor or manager who permits and encourages upward mobility builds a motivated and productive staff.

Legal Considerations

Employment policies concerning the promotion of employees must comply with Title VII of the Civil Rights Act of 1964, as amended. Thus, promotion policies should be written to ensure that they do not discriminate against any employee because of race, color, religion, gender, national origin, disability, or age.

The *Uniform Guidelines on Employee Selection Procedures*[14] requires that tests used to select employees for promotion be predictive of or significantly correlated with important elements of job performance. Under the regulations issued by the Office of Federal Contract Compliance Programs, posting job openings by the employer is an important part of any affirmative action program designed to upgrade female and minority employees and to ensure that people with disabilities have equal employment opportunities.

Why Have a Promotion Policy?

Employees are more motivated to perform effectively and efficiently if managers and supervisors support a policy of promotion from within. The policy should establish the guidelines to follow when a position opens. All promotion decisions should be based on merit, work record, and selected examinations. Seniority should be considered only if two or more applicants for the same job are equally qualified. A time limit for accepting applications should be set. Job bids from the staff must be received by the appropriate person before the deadline date to be considered for an open position.

When promoting employees, your medical group runs the risk of the employee being unable to satisfactorily perform the job. For this reason, a promoted employee should serve a six-month training period. If the employee fails to perform the new job satisfactorily, your policy should state whether s/he should be reinstated to the former position or to a comparable position, if one exists.

Promotion is a morale builder and an inducement for others interested in growth and advancement. All efforts should be made to ensure that promoted employees remain on the job for at least six months to reduce turnover and compensate for the training period.

Transfers

Transfers are another good way to fill vacant positions. You should have a written policy that explains your group's philosophy about transfers. The transfer policy should establish eligibility requirements. Three criteria that should be considered when deciding whether an employee should be transferred are:

- The employee's ability to perform the new job;
- Whether his or her performance was satisfactory in the former job; and
- The salary grade of the new position compared to the former one.

Usually, an employee will accept a transfer to a new position at the same salary, assuming that the same skills or previously acquired skills are used. In all cases, management should retain the right to transfer employees, regardless of whether they agree with the transfer. Sometimes an employee has difficulty performing his or her present duties because of personality differences with the present supervisor, the working dynamics of the department, or a conflict with another staff member. Under these circumstances, management might consider transferring the employee to another position to determine whether the supervisor, staff, or surroundings are the cause of the work difficulties, rather than a lack of ability to perform the duties. In this way, turnover can be reduced, and ultimately the employee is happier in his or her new position. In other cases, the employee may feel s/he needs a change of atmosphere, an opportunity to advance in a different type of work, or a different set of working hours that may be available in a different department. It is in your group's best interest to try to accommodate an employee's request for a transfer.

Why Have a Transfer Policy?

The right to transfer or reassign employees when reasonably necessary is considered a management function.

In the absence of a written policy establishing transfer procedures, employees will often attempt to negotiate a transfer directly with a supervisor rather than with the appropriate manager. The decisions about whether to approve a transfer should be based on input from everyone affected by the transfer and coordinated by the appropriate managers or an HR representative.

If an employee refuses to be transferred, s/he should be subject to disciplinary action for insubordination. Under no circumstance, however, should an employee be transferred as a disciplinary measure. Any disciplinary action related to insubordination should be described in your medical group's policies and procedures manual and be appropriate to the offense. In addition, frequent employee requests for transfers should not be permitted. This recurring activity is a clear warning that potential performance problems exist.

Temporary transfers may be necessary to meet temporary work overloads, address a staff shortage, avoid overtime, and prevent the need to hire temporary help. A transfer may include a change in work days, hours, or location.

Retention and Motivation

The ability to retain and motivate your most talented employees is directly related to the success of your group practice. The cost of recruiting and training new employees is easily double that of a departing employee's salary. Because of the shortages of qualified applicants in many health care fields, retaining your top talent is crucial to your group's success. Your group practice should establish a culture that promotes employee involvement and encourages top talent to stay with the practice for the long run. Your goal should be to become an "employer of choice" in your community.

Many talented employees seek to work for a high-performance and well-run group practice. They want an opportunity to grow within their jobs, increase their responsibilities, and obtain promotions. Top talent wants competitive pay and fringe benefits based on a performance- and merit-based reward system. Motivation starts at the top of your group practice. Motivated managers have motivated employees. Management should be proactive in anticipating any dissatisfaction in their top employees. To motivate and retain your employees, your group practice should find out what employees want, and then determine either how to give it to them or how they can earn it.

Elements for retaining and motivating top talent are :

- Employee engagement;
- Continuing education; and
- Competitive rewards and incentives.

Employee Engagement

Organizations with engaged employees are successful, productive, and cost-effective. Labor is the largest expense in most group practices. Finding a way to retain and motivate your top employees increases productivity and profitability. In a recent Gallup poll, businesses in the top 24 percent of employee engagement had less turnover and higher profitability, revenues, and percentages of customer loyalty. The correlation between employee engagement and productivity is strong.

Engagement begins by providing your employees with everything and anything, within reason, that they need to do their jobs and be successful. Employees should have all the materials they need within arm's reach to be as productive as possible. Your supervisors should be sure that new hires have the necessary resources to start working in their new positions immediately and to continue their work throughout the year.

Your group practice should clearly communicate to all employees what is expected of them, what the vision of the group practice is, what the group practice values, and how the group practice measures success. Employees cannot be engaged or productive if they do not know what is expected from them and how they will be evaluated. Your group practice's vision should be shared by all top-level managers, and you should encourage your employees to help the group practice achieve its vision. Lastly, employees become motivated and engaged when the rewards they earn truly mean something. Getting to know each of your employee's personality and behavioral traits and providing employee-specific rewards will increase productivity, engagement, motivation, and retention.

Many people want to feel that their skills are being used to the optimal level in their jobs. Managers should be aware of which employees have what skills and place them in job functions that optimize those skills. Employees should also be given responsibilities that they find challenging but not overly stressful.

Continuing Education

Providing continuing education opportunities adds to an employee's job satisfaction. Continuing education can be used to train your most talented employees to become the next generation of managers, or it can be used as a reward incentive. Continuing education is a must for many of your employees to keep their technical skills current. However, offering continuing education programs to noncertified or nonlicensed employees is a good practice for enhancing motivation and retention.

Competitive Rewards and Incentives

The goal of incentive and reward programs is to positively reinforce the desired on-the-job behavior, improve employee morale, and contribute to employee retention.

The benefits of offering rewards and incentives are that it:

- Stimulates a higher level of performance;
- Recognizes employee contributions;
- Creates a positive work environment;
- Positively affects employee retention;
- Creates and identifies mentors;
- Develops, improves, and sustains morale;
- Establishes a competitive advantage; and
- Provides better service to patients.

Group practices with a highly participatory work environment that recognizes and rewards top performance outperform those practices that do not. Some may rationalize that salaried employees who earn a competitive wage are paid enough, and that salary should be a sufficient source of motivation and recognition. In reality, money does little to encourage employees to do their best work or exceed expectations.

Extra effort and increased commitment are more a function of how workers are treated than what they are paid. Studies dating as far back as the 1940s support this assertion, with employees consistently ranking factors such as interesting work, supervisors' appreciation, job security, and participation in decision making as being more important than their salaries. Although money can be effective in some situations, it usually provides only a brief stimulus, whereas personal recognition and appreciation have longer-term positive effects. Today, reward incentive programs are replacing the traditional monetary reward systems of the past.

There are two distinct types of incentive programs: those initiated by the group practice and those contingent on performance. Although performance-based programs are used less often by group practices, they are often more effective and less costly.

Group practice–initiated incentives are provided to the entire staff and thus do not reward high-level performance or directly contribute to the bottom line. These types of incentives are important for boosting morale and showing general appreciation, but they do not focus on specific, goal-oriented behavior to motivate employees. Christmas bonuses, for example, are not a reward for performance.

Other examples of group practice–initiated incentives include giving an employee flowers on his or her first day of work and giving turkeys and other food gifts during the holidays. Many employees celebrate staff birthdays with cards, flowers, cakes, small gifts, or potluck lunches. Other practices hold staff parties, picnics, or a planning retreat away from the office. Some employers pay for an overnight stay, and then leave the second day free for fun.

At the opposite end of the spectrum are incentives contingent on performance, which directly affects the practice's overall performance and bottom line. They identify positive behaviors and are tied to the group practice's mission or specific project goals.

Within a practice's incentive program are rewards, which are categorized as formal or informal. Traditionally, most reward programs were highly structured and used to recognize above-average employee performance or milestone years of service. These types of rewards tend to be more impersonal and infrequent. Rewards that are used repeatedly lose their effectiveness over time. Most of these formal programs create a special time when outstanding accomplishments of staff are communicated and celebrated by the entire staff.

Group practices are increasingly offering informal reward and recognition programs, which demonstrate spontaneous appreciation of top-level performance. Not only are these programs inexpensive, but they can also be quickly implemented and easily maintained. The philosophy is that it's the little things that count the most. Informal rewards can be categorized as monetary or nonmonetary.

Examples of monetary rewards are:

- Creating a gift closet from which top performers can select items such as coffee mugs, pen sets, movies, and music;

- Distributing tickets to sporting events, movies, concerts, or cultural events;

- Subsidizing gym memberships;
- Providing a thank-you gift basket to an employee and his or her family who worked particularly long hours on a special project;
- Giving gift certificates;
- Taking top performers to a midday movie of their choice;
- Sending employees to professional organization meetings;
- Approving educational expenses and tuition reimbursements;
- Scheduling shopping sprees and giving envelopes with cash to spend;
- Giving vouchers for professional income tax preparation;
- Giving spa services;
- Arranging for nights out on the town, including dinner and a movie; and
- Providing breakfast or lunch on busy days.

Some group practices structure rewards around the family by subsidizing diaper services, in-home tutoring, or summer day camps. Some practices hire their staff's teenage children for administrative support during school vacations.

Monetary rewards need not involve large amounts of money; any amount from fifty to several hundred dollars can be effective. If you use monetary rewards, separate them from the employee's regular paycheck; otherwise they may be overlooked or undervalued.

Remember that gifts up to $25, such as flowers and gift certificates, are tax deductible. Achievement rewards such as televisions, small appliances, jewelry, crystal, and china are deductible up to $400. Be sure to consult with your tax attorney or accountant since tax laws change often.

Examples of nonmonetary rewards are:

- Putting gold stars or other recognition on employees' name badges;
- Giving time-off certificates;

- Preparing a practice or department yearbook featuring individuals and team accomplishments and photos from staff events;

- Letting top performers work flexible hours;

- Giving employees more prestigious titles when appropriate;

- Posting special achievement and thank-you letters;

- Creating a wall of fame featuring top employees' photos;

- Recognizing contributions by assigning a special parking spot;

- Highlighting top performers and their accomplishments in your practice's newsletter;

- Holding staff thank-you meetings, at which everyone thanks someone else for something they accomplished;

- Sending news releases to the local media, detailing staff's accomplishments and awards;

- Featuring top performers in the practice's printed marketing materials; and

- Washing an employee's car during lunch.

Rewarding your employees with extra time off is a very popular reward that oftentimes is valued more than money. Another benefit is that the group practice does not have to pay higher taxes because of higher salaries. Variations on how to award time off include adding time to a holiday or weekend.

How best to establish an incentive program that fits your group practice's needs depends on the practice's size and its philosophy on compensation and incentives. You start by identifying employee wants and needs through such means as employee surveys or focus groups. If the practice already has an incentive program in place, this is a good time to ask employees if the current program is still meaningful and how it can be improved. From this information, you can develop realistic goals for the program and identify what levels of achievement will be recognized. See Exhibit 3.

Taking time to educate managers and staff about your rewards program, as well as getting their support, is critical to the success of the program. Share the thinking behind the program, the importance of recognition, and the role the program plays in helping the practice achieve its goals.

Schedule separate training and orientation programs for the management team and the rest of the staff, as each group plays a different role and has different interests in the rewards program. Explain how the program works, and then manage expectations for how performance rewards are recognized and rewarded before the implementation date. Once the program is up and running, communicate its results regularly.

Meaningful recognition should come first from the immediate supervisor, then the management team, physicians, and top administrator, as appropriate. No matter how busy your schedule, this is not the time for delegation – that is, never ask an associate to recognize the employee or write a note of thanks on your behalf. Part of the value of the recognition is that it comes from a manager who took his or her own time to express appreciation for a job well done. When recognizing an outstanding employee, highlight how his or her behavior affected the supervisor, the team, the department, and/or the practice.

Pitfalls to avoid are:

- Offering one-size-fits-all incentives;
- Offering insincere flattery and exaggerating employees' accomplishments;
- Using incentives as a substitute for paying competitive wages;
- Giving only cash rewards;
- Overlooking employees who deserve rewards;
- Structuring performance targets that are difficult to understand;
- Sending notes of praise that also contain criticism;

EXHIBIT 3

Reward Guidelines

Reward guidelines focus on recognizing employee performance frequently and personally, through both formal and informal means. The following tips can assist you as you develop your rewards programs:

1. Design rewards according to the group's culture. Rewards and incentives should be in line with the practice's culture and value system.

2. Link rewards to business goals. Rewards should be closely aligned to practice goals and support the practice's overall strategy and mission.

3. Allow for flexibility. Be flexible enough to respond to changes in the practice's strategic direction and staff needs. Give supervisors latitude in how they recognize outstanding achievements, and encourage on-the-spot recognition.

4. Keep the program simple and easy to understand. Communicate the structure and benefits of the reward program so that managers and staff can easily understand and embrace it.

5. Match the reward to employees' performance outcomes. Employees need to understand exactly why they are being rewarded. Otherwise, they will only experience a short-term glow without lasting impact.

6. Be consistent in how you identify outstanding performance. Avoid favoritism among employees, and recognize everyone who produces targeted behaviors. Inconsistent feedback sends confusing messages and contributes to low morale.

7. Tailor the reward to the recipient. Ask recipients, as well as their colleagues, what rewards they value most. Then let employees choose among several options. Avoid rewards that might embarrass an employee, and be sensitive to individual needs and personalities.

EXHIBIT 3 *(Continued)*
Reward Guidelines

8. Make recognition timely. Timely and equitably distributed rewards are essential to stimulating outstanding performance. Very little time should lapse between the desired behavior and the corresponding recognition. The value of timely recognition is its immediacy and the likelihood that it will lead to repeated behavior.

9. Reward frequently. Allow employees to build on achievements and continue improving by using small perks on a regular basis, thereby creating lasting value.

10. Review and revise your rewards program regularly. Solicit ongoing feedback from staff, making adjustments as necessary and communicating those adjustments in a timely manner.

11. Track employee achievements. Include in employees' files a record of outstanding performance and recognition. Notify employees' family members of special recognition, too.

- Using the same rewards repeatedly so that they lose their effectiveness;

- Telling someone they're doing a good job but failing to mention specific behaviors; and

- Giving credit for the achievements of other staff members.

The challenge today is not only to revamp outdated incentive and retention programs and design new ones, but also to continually implement, manage, and evaluate their results. Successfully implementing these programs can help your group practice retain a more motivated, productive work force while making a significant contribution to the practice's bottom line.

Employee Conduct

Certain rules and regulations governing employee behavior are necessary for the orderly operation of your group practice and for the protection and safety of your employees and patients. These rules and regulations usually establish your code of conduct for employees to follow. The rules should communicate your sincere interest to protect, assist, and guide employees in performing their job duties and responsibilities, especially in how they interact with patients. A code of conduct can help guide your employees' behavior and ensure the proper image for your medical group.

A code of conduct should state what is expected of employees in general terms. Regulating employee conduct is a matter that should be handled with the utmost sensitivity. Employees should be treated with respect and dignity, in recognition of individual worth. Most organizations shy away from specific rules that may be too restrictive or unnecessary. A code of conduct should clearly define prohibited conduct. Should the need for disciplinary action arise, your decisions will be more readily accepted by employees if a comprehensive conduct policy has been established and communicated to your employees.

Although most organizations have written employment policies and procedures concerning employee conduct, the scope of these policies varies greatly. The subject covers many areas and depends on your philosophy. Your group should consider establishing your own code of employee conduct, using the list in Exhibit 4 as a guide.

Why Have an Employee Conduct Policy?

The employee conduct policy is a code of ethical conduct and prescribed behavior. It should clearly specify types of prohibited conduct and indicate that disciplinary action is taken for violations. You should consistently follow and enforce the policy. Employees usually see through a policy that is not taken seriously by managers and supervisors. How individuals act typically depends on how the people at the top act. The conduct policy should be well communicated to staff.

EXHIBIT 4
Elements to Consider When Establishing an Employee Conduct Code

- Absenteeism – Excessive absenteeism should be prohibited. All absences must be reported to the supervisor prior to starting time.

- Attitude – Employees should be courteous, friendly, helpful, and prompt in dealing with patients and co-workers. Their attitude reflects your practice and influences the patient's opinions of the practice.

- Bulletin boards – Posting, altering, or removing any material on the bulletin boards or online posting sites, unless authorized, is prohibited.

- Business travel – An employee who is authorized to use his or her car for business is expected to carry adequate amounts of liability insurance. The medical group's insurance is secondary to the driver's personal insurance coverage. Employees must also have a valid driver's license and proof of insurance when driving for business purposes.

- Cameras – Using cameras, including those in cell phones, within the medical group facilities by employees or visitors is not permitted without authorization or prior permission.

- Carelessness and negligence – Careless or negligent acts during working hours or on medical group property are prohibited.

- Charity drives – Employees should be encouraged to participate in charitable functions, but this is not mandatory.

- Check cashing – In cases of emergency, personal checks may be cashed by the accounting or bookkeeping departments.

- Collections and gifts – Collections taken for gifts, activities, parties, and so on are kept to a minimum. Participation is strictly voluntary. Management approval must be obtained.

- Community emergencies – Employees who serve as members of volunteer groups, including emergency aid units, air search, fire fighting, mountain rescue, and underwater search teams may be granted time off when assisting in community emergencies.

- Competitors – An employee is prohibited from working directly or indirectly for a competitor of the medical group. This includes self-employment ventures.

EXHIBIT 4 *(Continued)*
Elements to Consider When Establishing an Employee Conduct Code

- Computers and Internet – Rules about access to computers, authorization to use computers, and control of data should appear in your operating procedures.

- Confidential information – The unauthorized disclosure of any medical group or patient information that could be damaging to the group's and individual's interests is prohibited.

- Conflict of interest – Employees must refrain from engaging in any activity or practice that conflicts with the interests of the group or its patients, such as using the business relationship for personal gain.

- Co-worker relations – Employees should be nondiscriminating, fair, and friendly in dealing with fellow employees. Cooperation ensures pleasant working conditions. A good attitude toward fellow employees enhances the efficiency of the group.

- Damage to information, records, or property – Damage, loss, destruction, and any attempt to conceal defective information, records, and property are prohibited.

- Decorum – Professional conduct is expected at all times by all employees. Conversations should be in low tones and pertain only to business matters.

- Discrimination – The medical group is an equal opportunity employer. Discrimination in any form is prohibited.

- Disorderly conduct – Disorderly conduct during working hours is prohibited. This includes fighting, scuffling, horseplay, and threatening or abusing other employees.

- Dress code – Employees required to wear a uniform must be in uniform at all times while on duty. The employee is responsible for keeping it clean. Employees whose jobs require street clothing should be well groomed and use good judgment in choosing apparel. They should dress in a neat and businesslike manner. Management may authorize casual dress days on occasion. Personal cleanliness and clean apparel are expected.

EXHIBIT 4 *(Continued)*
Elements to Consider When Establishing an Employee Conduct Code

- Encouraging violation of work rules – Encouraging, bribing, coercing, inciting, or otherwise inducing any employee to engage in any practice violating the medical group's work rules is prohibited.

- Explosives – Possessing explosives and other dangerous or hazardous materials in any form during working hours and on medical group property at any time is prohibited.

- Falsification of time cards – Falsifying time cards, punching another employee's time card, or having one's time card punched by another is prohibited.

- Financial obligations – Employees are expected to meet financial obligations and avoid discredit to themselves or the medical group.

- Firearms – Possessing firearms or weapons of any nature during working hours or on medical group property is prohibited.

- Fraudulent statements – Fraudulent statements that attempt to destroy or injure are prohibited.

- Gambling – Gambling during working hours or on group property is prohibited.

- Garnishments – Employees are expected to meet their financial obligations and avoid garnishments that could discredit themselves or the group.

- Gossip – Engaging in idle or malicious talk is discouraged.

- Gratuities and gifts – Employees must refuse to accept any compensation or gift that might result in preferential treatment of people, businesses, or organizations. Also, employees should discourage patients from offering gifts and gratuities.

- Housekeeping – Employees should keep their work area clean, neat, and orderly.

- Identification badges – Badges must be worn at all times while on the group's property. Lending a badge to another person is prohibited.

- Insubordination – Refusing to comply with supervisory orders concerning job-related matters is prohibited.

EXHIBIT 4 *(Continued)*

Elements to Consider When Establishing an Employee Conduct Code

- Intent to harm – Destroying property, inflicting bodily injury, and attempting destruction or injury are prohibited.

- Leaving work – Preparing to leave work before the end of a shift is prohibited.

- Loafing and loitering – Employees are expected to work each hour for which they are paid. Loafing, loitering, and engaging in unauthorized visiting during working time is prohibited.

- Loss of property, records, or information – Willful loss of, damage to, unauthorized use of, and destruction of property, records, or information are prohibited.

- Maintenance of equipment and machines – Employees should keep equipment and machines clean and in good working condition. Problems should be reported to a supervisor.

- Media relations – If contacted by the press, employees should refer these contacts to medical group management immediately.

- Narcotics and alcohol – Unauthorized use, sale, or possession of non-prescription drugs or alcohol on medical group premises is prohibited.

- Nepotism – No person can be hired in a regular full- or part-time position who has a relative working as a supervisor in that department.

- Offensive language – Offensive, abusive, or improper language during working hours is prohibited.

- Patient/employee relations – In relationships with patients and the public, employees should use good manners, patience, understanding, and respect.

- Personal belongings – Safeguarding, replacing, or repairing personal property that has been lost, stolen, or damaged is the responsibility of the employee. Employees are discouraged from bringing valuable items to work.

- Personal loans – The medical group does not take responsibility or assist in recovering money loaned by one employee to another. The best practice is not to make loans.

EXHIBIT 4 *(Continued)*
Elements to Consider When Establishing an Employee Conduct Code

- Personal mail – Due to the large volume of incoming mail, employees are prohibited from using the medical group as a personal mailing address, either through the postal service, the fax machine, or e-mail. Medical group letterhead stationery and equipment are used for business purposes only.

- Personal projects – Any personal project that uses the group's equipment and materials must be approved by management.

- Personal visitors – Personal visitors interfere with work and disrupt other employees. Visitors and personal calls are not to be received during working hours.

- Pets – Pets are not allowed in the medical group facilities at any time.

- Political activity – Individuals engaging in political activities must ensure that such activities do not interfere with their responsibilities to the medical group.

- Professional organizations – Salaried employees may participate in professional organizations relating specifically to their jobs or specialties. Professional subscriptions and dues may be paid by the company with prior approval from the medical group management.

- Property pass – Any person removing property from the medical group must obtain a property pass from a supervisor.

- Reading – Personal reading during working time is prohibited.

- Sleeping – Sleeping during working time is prohibited.

- Slowdowns and idleness – Willfully holding back, slowing down, hindering, or limiting production in any way is prohibited.

- Smoking – Employees may not smoke in areas where smoking is prohibited.

- Solicitations – Solicitations that interfere with an employee's patient care responsibilities are prohibited.

- Stealing – Stealing is prohibited.

- Telephone use – Personal phone calls are to be kept to a minimum.

> EXHIBIT 4 *(Continued)*
> ## Elements to Consider When Establishing an Employee Conduct Code
>
> ■ Threats – Threats or intimidation by any employee is prohibited.
>
> ■ Unauthorized possession of the medical group's possessions – Unauthorized possession, removal, or use of any company property or equipment is prohibited.
>
> ■ Voting – Employees should use personal leave to vote. When this is not possible, a supervisor must approve time off to vote without loss of pay.
>
> ■ Workplace harassment – Workplace harassment including sexual harassment is prohibited. Harassment ranges from offensive remarks to annoyances and distractions to deliberate intimidation, threats, and demands of physical acts. Harassment is not tolerated, and disciplinary action may be taken, including termination.

◼ Conflict Resolution

Establishing effective employee relations and appropriate conflict resolution programs are necessary to work toward common goals. The word *team* is overused in health care – it conveys the expectation that everyone will work together to accomplish a common purpose. Often, employees and departments experience conflicts that thwart the attainment of high performance. When this happens, the supervisor needs to get involved and talk with the employees one-on-one or in groups to identify the problems and determine a resolution. Sometimes an objective third party may need to get involved if issues are plagued with cultural or historical resistance or the process of change isn't supported by the physicians. Also, another party may need to get involved if the conflict is between the employee and supervisor. Differences in problem-solving styles, information processing, and communication can create conflicts that, if not resolved soon after identification, may produce disastrous results.

■ Personnel Policy

The personnel policy should state which representative will resolve the issue. It may be the HR representative, the medical practice executive, or an employee and labor relations consultant, or, if the practice is unionized, the union steward. This person will meet with the employee, supervisor, or both, as may be appropriate to the chain of command, to help in resolving their differences. This representative can provide advice on matters of policy interpretation, rights of management and employees, and information on the formal grievance process.

The personnel policy may have a statement on protection against retaliation of the employee for exercising his or her rights under the arbitration process. There may be time limits on the process to facilitate speedy resolution of the problem while providing appropriate time to collect, prepare, and present information. For example, if the employee fails to follow the time limits, the issue may be deemed to be resolved to the employee's satisfaction. If the medical practice fails to follow specific time limits, the employee may take the complaint to a higher level of resolution. Personnel policies should reflect current federal, state, and local employment laws.

Policy Interpretation for Grievance Procedures

For all disciplinary action, policy interpretation is a human resources responsibility. The disciplinary action or progressive discipline process is meant to give appropriate feedback to the employee in a formal way. This constructive feedback for desired results is meant to provide the employee with measurable accomplishments, instill individual accountability and responsibility, and facilitate the desired behavior. The supervisor can serve as a mentor, coach, and facilitator of the process and help the employee understand the desired results.

If the communication requires multiple areas of behavior change, the supervisor may choose to give the employee a performance improvement plan (PIP). This tool focuses on below-average or substandard performance and provides an action plan for needed change. The plan is time specific and allows the employee to receive periodic feedback. For example, an employee may receive a PIP for inappropriate interactions with patients. The PIP would provide the employee with customer service training and weekly feedback sessions between the supervisor and employee on improvement in the desired results. Failure to achieve desired results can lead to additional disciplinary action up to and including termination. The PIP's intent is to help the employee be successful and shepherd the process along the way.

◼ Mediation

Mediation allows the employer and employee to troubleshoot issues and come to positive relations. It allows problems to be dealt with promptly and provides an opportunity to address a problem before it escalates into an unworkable issue. Usually, mediation will move away from blame or judgment and allow a win/win situation, as opposed to a win/lose situation. The two parties, not the mediator, control the situation and the outcome. Mediation can be used prior to a formal grievance process, such as arbitration. Using mediation, however, does not waive one's right to use a formal grievance process if the parties cannot reach a satisfactory outcome through mediation.

In mediation, a professional mediator contacts the two parties involved and seeks to achieve agreement. Usually, each party meets individually with a mediator first to identify and discuss the concerns. The mediator will keep all information from these sessions confidential. Then the mediator will bring the two parties together to discuss the concerns, and will work toward a win/win outcome. Sometimes a second session may be required, depending on the complexity of the issue. If the two parties reach an agreement, the mediator will work with them to create a written agreement listing the specific components of the agreement, which both parties will sign. Usually, these agreements do not change existing medical practice policies or union contracts.

■ Arbitration

Nonbinding arbitration is a way of avoiding disputes because it provides a written guide on the practice used in employee grievances. The purpose of the arbitration policy is to establish a procedure for the fair, orderly, and speedy resolution of disputes that sometimes arise between management and employees. The policy will state to whom it applies (e.g., all members, unclassified employees) and how the policy is used. An employee may use the procedure to review an alleged violation of the medical practice's policy or rules pertaining to employment.

In a nonbinding arbitration process, two parties give a dispute to a neutral person to determine an advisory or nonbinding decision, meaning that neither party is required to accept the opinion. In the process, the two groups have input into the selection of the person arbitrating. Nonbinding arbitration is used when the parties want a quick dispute resolution, prefer a third-party decision maker, and want more control over the decision-making process if not resolved. In binding arbitration, both parties present a dispute to an impartial arbitrator to determine a binding decision. The parties have the ability to decide who serves as the arbitrator. Binding arbitration is appropriate when the parties want a neutral third party to decide the outcome of the dispute and avoid a formal trial. The parties do not retain control over how their dispute is resolved and cannot appeal the arbitrator's decision.

■ Employee Grievance Procedures[15]

Initially, there should be an attempt at an informal resolution of complaints. Regular communication between the practice managers and employees reduces the need for a more formal review and is in the mutual best interest of the medical practice and employees. Written resources materials, handouts, and guides should always be available to help management communicate information with employees. An employee who has a work-related problem should bring it to the medical practice executive's attention with the intent of resolving the problem. In a timely manner, management should discuss the concern with the employee with an effort to resolve the issue. If informal attempts at resolution are not satisfactory, employees may use a formal grievance process.

Listening to employees is key to ensuring excellent performance. Active listening will help to identify whether any issues or concerns are preventing the employee from performing the expected job duties. Early identification of problems can avoid serious problems later. If, through active listening, a supervisor recognizes that a problem exists that requires a higher level of problem solving or counseling, the supervisor needs to recognize his or her limitations and refer the employee to either the Human Resource Department or, if offered, an Employee Assistance Program (EAP) to help the employee sort through personal issues that are inhibiting acceptable performance levels.

Progressive Discipline

What does discipline mean to an organization? Corrective action strives to provide feedback to an employee to correct a behavior. Progressive discipline sets parameters on which behaviors are unacceptable and how the negative behaviors requiring change will be communicated with the employee. Large medical groups usually have a progressive discipline process that clearly establishes expectations and consequences of those behaviors if not met. The discipline process may be different for the staff and physicians. The purpose of having a constructive discipline process is to establish guidelines that will ensure an environment that is efficient, productive, and orderly to provide standards and rules governing performance and a procedure for consistent, nondiscriminatory application of the rules with the intent of providing quality patient care. The policy does not apply to employees who are in their new hire period or per diem or temporary employees. The personnel policy applies to part-time and full-time regular status employees.

Progressive discipline must be fair, consistent, well understood, and timely. Lack of a consistent process to administer discipline may ultimately lead to a disgruntled employee filing a lawsuit. A progressive discipline program provides the employee with feedback that clearly outlines unacceptable behavior and the consequences if this behavior is not changed. Usually progressive discipline involves a verbal warning followed by a written warning. If behavior doesn't change, a suspension or final written warning is the next level of discipline. Ultimately, if behavior doesn't improve, the employee may be terminated. Some behaviors may warrant a progressive level, and other behaviors may warrant more, or may skip a step and move into a higher level of discipline. For example, chronic tardiness would go through progressive discipline, whereas stealing money would result in immediate termination or suspension, pending an administrative investigation. Employees must understand that there is a process for discipline and consequences to bad behavior.

If a union is present in a practice, the union's progressive discipline process may require a union representative to be present with the union employee and manager when progressive discipline is administered.

Recorded Conference

For rule infractions considered less serious, a recorded conference may be the first step in the corrective action process. It consists of a verbal conference with, at a minimum, the employee and supervisor and will be documented in writing and placed in the employee's personnel file. Examples of behavior for which a recorded conference may be initiated as the first step of the correction action process include:

- Work area absence without permission (e.g., leaving work without clocking out);

- Extended lunch time or breaks without permission (e.g., taking a 30-minute break instead of a 15-minute break);

- Loitering during scheduled work time or during off-duty hours (e.g., staying in work area after shift and creating disturbances with employees);

- Smoking or eating in unauthorized areas (e.g., eating in surgical area that is a sterile environment);

- Conducting personal business on work premises (e.g., selling products during work time);

- Violation of parking rules (e.g., parking in a "no parking" or "patients only" zone for the duration of a work shift);

- Improper attire or appearance (e.g., wearing jeans or denim when not part of the dress code);

- Inefficiency or incompetence in work duties performed (e.g., failing to perform job duty during work shift);

- Unauthorized telephone use (e.g., making long-distance or extensive personal calls without permission); or

- Attendance problems (e.g., showing up late for work without prior notice or permission).

Written Corrective Action

The written corrective action is a document summarizing the performance problem or incident detrimental to the customer, inability to follow established policy, or the failure to respond to supervision. A written corrective action serves as notice that continued infractions will not be tolerated and/or that performance must improve to meet expectations. Examples of behavior for which a written corrective action may be initiated as the first step of the corrective active process include:

- Inappropriate treatment or behavior toward a customer;

- Conduct prejudicial to the best interest of the medical group;

- Careless, indifferent, or negligent job performance, including unsafe or unsanitary practices;

- Careless, neglectful, unauthorized, or improper use of company property or equipment;

- Collecting money or accepting gratuities for personal use;

- Failure of good behavior or neglect of duty; or

- Repeated or chronic infractions with no evident improvement in performance or conduct.

Suspension or Final Written Corrective Action

An unpaid suspension or final written corrective action in lieu of suspension may occur when performance continues to be detrimental to customer satisfaction or where a serious performance problem exists. Suspensions should be scheduled at a time as close to the infraction as possible but also so that patient care and consistency of service do not suffer. Depending on the seriousness of the incident or behavior, the employee may receive a suspension or final written corrective action as the first step of the corrective action process.

Examples of behavior warranting suspension include possession, use, or sale of alcohol, narcotics, or controlled substances on the medical group premises, or reporting to work under the influence of alcohol or narcotics, usually evidenced by one or more of the following behaviors:

- Inability to perform assigned work;

- Presentation of undesirable attributes (e.g., hygiene, attitude, uncooperativeness);

- Insubordination or refusal to perform a reasonable assignment after having been instructed by a supervisor to do so;

- Sleeping on the job;

- Disorderly conduct;

- Failure to conform to professional standards; or

- Any other critical failure of good behavior or serious neglect of duty.

Termination

Termination may occur as the final step in the corrective action process. Termination of an employee is never an easy task, but it is a necessary one if the employee does not consistently follow the medical groups' policies and procedures. Termination may occur for serious offenses or for continued performance problems impacting the customer. Examples of behavior where immediate termination may be initiated as the first step of corrective action include:

- Threat of or actual physical or verbal abuse of patients, visitors, employees;

- Inappropriate treatment of any patient for any reason;

- Falsification of any official medical group records (e.g., medical records);

- Illegal or dishonest act;

- Damage or theft of property;

- Absence from work without justifiable reason or, in some practices, without reporting off for two (or more, depending on the practice's variables) consecutive working days;

- Unauthorized possession, use, copying, or revealing of confidential information regarding patients, employees, or medical group activity;

- Unwelcome sexual advances, requests for sexual favors, or other verbal or physical conduct of a sexual nature with an employee, visitor, or patient;

- Harassment in any form, including that based on race, gender, religion, or national origin, which includes offensive jokes, ridicule, or racial, religious, sexual, or ethnic slurs;

- Improper use of leave of absence;

- Conviction of a felony relevant to the employee's position;

- Solicitation and/or distribution of literature (e.g., pornography, political campaigns, etc.); or

- Any other gross neglect of good behavior or gross neglect of duty.

Employee Assistance Program

In today's changing workplace environment, the medical practice executive is expected to provide more services with fewer dollars. Employees are expected to do more tasks and handle stressful situations professionally. This stress may cause worry, confusion, doubt, and even sickness. Dealing with prolonged stress may cause fatigue, depression, anger, and anxiety, which may lead to defensiveness, inappropriate behavior, and co-worker conflict. Although some worry and anxiety is normal, sometimes these emotions can become problematic and impact employee productivity, lower employee morale, and foster poor outcomes. An Employee Assistance Program helps the employee stay on track and provides coping mechanisms to perform better in a state of uncertainty.

An EAP is a medical practice resource that uses a comprehensive program of counseling services for employees and/or their dependents to help improve employee and workplace effectiveness. It provides confidential, third-party counseling and work/life services to employees in an off-site setting, and its effectiveness is through its efforts toward prevention, identification, and resolution of employee personal problems that impact employee productivity. EAP services may be provided by the employer's own EAP or provided through an external agency. The EAP is not a mandated employee benefit, yet it can be very beneficial in reducing employee risk, cutting costs for recruitment of new employees, and improving employee productivity. Employees may use an EAP for counseling or further referrals for financial counseling (e.g., bankruptcy, money management, gambling), family issues (e.g., death, divorce, separation), domestic violence (e.g., spousal or child abuse), alcohol and substance abuse, mental health issues (e.g., depression, suicidal ideation, phobias), and family law (e.g., adoption, custody, restraining orders). The medical practice executive may use an EAP to help employees better address issues that impact poor performance, provide an on-site counselor in case of a traumatic event (e.g., employee death), or provide on-site training to handle employee issues more effectively.

An EAP may be needed by an employee as a further condition of employment. If the employer believes that the employee cannot continue working in the medical practice without EAP services, then it becomes a mandatory referral. However, most EAP services are sought by the employee voluntarily. EAP services usually are available to all part-time and full-time employees, regardless of employment position.

EAP and Counseling

Counseling for Emotional Issues

On a basic level, it is important for an employee to have good emotional health. An EAP provides support to employees and helps them to address emotional issues. The physician, medical practice executive, or HR director is not a trained therapist. When it is determined that the dialogue with an employee is moving from sharing feelings to needing help in managing emotional issues, an EAP referral should be made. The staff is not equipped to handle professional counseling issues and should not attempt to provide such counseling.

Family/Marital Counseling

Numerous family issues may prevent an employee from completing work accurately or being on time for the medical practice. Persistent feelings of dissatisfaction may impact the workplace and create disruptions. Counseling can help to address problems with a child's behavior, school adjustment, or performance; difficulties with anger, hostility, or violence; family stress due to illness; stepfamilies dealing with stepchildren; and ex-spouses.

Financial Counseling

Employees may have financial problems that may distract them from their work and create decreased productivity. A troubled employee may distract other employees and ask for help from co-workers who are not qualified or have the skills necessary to help the employee. Typical financial areas may include issues with debt, money management, credit, and consumer and retirement planning.

Legal Counseling

Legal counseling can help the employee to address legal issues, clarify goals, find appropriate counsel, and address appropriate legal costs.

Career Counseling

Employees can get stuck in a rut or a job with no future. Career counseling can help the employee to gain help in career planning by addressing:

- How to conduct a self-assessment;
- How to address career advancement options;
- How to identify skill development opportunities;
- How to write a resume;
- How to respond in an interview;
- How to identify available continuing-education workshops; and
- How to cope with transitions in a job function or duty.

EAP and Potential Workplace Violence

According to the U.S. Bureau of Labor Statistics' Census of Fatal Occupational Injuries, there were 639 workplace homicides and 8,787 fatal work injuries in the United States in 2001.[16] The medical practice physicians and staff need to have the required skills to identify, prevent, minimize, and eliminate violent and aggressive behaviors. An EAP can help a medical practice to develop an effective program that brings management commitment and employee involvement together to create an environment that has a zero-tolerance policy on workplace violence.

EAP and Stress Management

Stress is neither good nor bad. It is how we manage stress that makes a difference on our bodies and minds. Negatively managing stress can create feelings of anger, depression, distrust, paranoia, and rejection; and result in health problems, such as high blood pressure, insomnia, rashes, headaches, and upset stomach. Any change can create stress in an employee's life, from a new job to managing a heavy workload to a death in the family to a new relationship. An EAP can help the employee to better manage stress, as opposed to eliminating stress.

EAP and Tolerance for No-Solution Situations

Sometimes an employee may be faced with a no-solution situation. An EAP can help the employee accept what can be changed, what cannot be changed, and what the employee can do to cope with these situations. As long as the employee is able to perform on the job based on the goals and expectations of the practice, the employee's success is based on his or her ability to handle stress constructively.

EAP and Age Discrimination

Change is inevitable in any medical practice. However, some workers stay in the same job for years. As new management or physicians come into a practice, they may institute change that is perceived as trying to eliminate the employee. Employee comments such as, "We've always done it this way, so why do we need to change" and "I'm too old to handle this kind of stress anymore" are indicators that the employee may perceive discrimination due to age. An EAP can help the employee address change in a positive way and help the employee see that age discrimination is not a factor when experiencing change.

EAP and Objectivity

An EAP is meant to provide an objective stance on an issue facing an employee. An EAP provides perspective and help where the employee may perceive that help is not available in the practice. For example, when a work-related issue arises, an employee may have difficulty handling criticism and indirect challenges of not performing. An EAP can help the employee to address these issues from an objective perspective.

During times of stress, an employee may turn employee issues away from self-review and focus energy on others. A common reaction is the sense that a policy interpretation and its follow-up are unfairly administered and applied. The EAP can provide an objective view and interpretation of those policies.

EAP and Substance Abuse/Impaired Physicians

Substance abuse may result in immediate termination or a mandatory referral to an EAP to seek necessary outpatient or/and inpatient treatment. Failure to seek mandatory treatment would result in immediate termination. A medical practice may have an "Impaired Physician Committee" to handle problems and concerns revolving around a physician's behavior or clinical competence during times of stress. The committee may address physician issues pertaining to substance abuse, health status, violence, sexual harassment, and mental status. All these issues may affect the physician's ability to care for the patient on a professional level.

■ Unions

The Wagner Act of 1935, otherwise known as the National Labor Relations Act (NLRA), was passed to protect employees' rights to unionize. The National Labor Relations Board (NLRB) was created to implement and enforce the NLRA. Numerous labor laws are currently in place; however, the Wagner Act marked the federal government's initial support for unionization and collective bargaining. The NLRB conducts elections to determine whether employees want union representation and also examines unfair labor practices by employers and unions. The act guarantees employees the right to self-organize, choose representation, and bargain collectively.

The NLRB must also make sure that employers do not discriminate against union members. Labor laws allow employees the right to unionize and to participate in strikes, picketing, and lockouts to have their demands met. Employee areas for consideration may include employees' amount of pay, pay methods, benefits, work hours, type of work performed, and qualifications required. It may also involve the workers' physical proximity and integration of tasks, the employer's supervisory or medical practice structure, and specific employee preferences. For example, union issues could involve the physical proximity of a group's work area to facilitate interaction among group members. If the work area was split across two floors of the same building, a union could see a negative impact on the group. The lack of proximity of the work spaces can create disintegration of work tasks and have a negative impact on the group's ability to perform its job, and therefore can be perceived as a burden on the work force.

Union-Free Work Force

For a medical practice to maintain a union-free workplace, it must be experienced in knowing how to combat union organization efforts. The medical practice executive's human resource function, along with legal counsel, can help the medical group address local union activity, organizing tactics and targets, early warning signs of union involvement, lawful employer countermeasures, effective personnel policies and practices, and the employer's legal rights in dealing with a union. The medical practice must provide its front-line supervisors and/or managers with the training necessary for lawful union avoidance. Managers must know what they can and cannot say about unions and unionization, and how they must communicate effectively with the employees they oversee. The practice executive should know how to effectively exercise the medical practice's legal rights due to assertive union campaigns, including how to lawfully communicate critical facts about collective bargaining, union dues, member obligations, strikes, and shutdowns to all employees; and how to deal with union campaign handouts, postings, speeches, and videos that are lawful. Usually, the consideration of a union is due to a lack of effective communication and problem solving with employees to address proper and effective employment practices.

Union Grievance Procedures

If a union has been established in a medical practice, the union contract will specify the grievance procedures. The process may be very similar to that for nonunion employees, although it is best to read both policies for confirmation.

Competitive Wages

Unions will dictate a competitive wage package and a schedule for wage increases. Commonly, the program does not provide merit increases, but rather a fixed increase for each union employee.

Communication Plan

When the union and the medical practice sign a contract, there is a communication plan to ensure that the union employees understand the agreement on the practice's procedures and policies.

■ Conclusion

Establishing effective employee relations and instituting conflict resolution programs are important functions in a medical practice. They provide for better communication between employee and employer and allow for opportunities to address grievances and employee issues. A medical practice executive should have a working knowledge of HR laws and regulations, grievance procedures, progressive discipline, and programs to help employees to be productive.

Summary

There is more to employee retention, discipline, and performance management than just annual performance evaluations. Individual performance goals and objectives should be set for each employee. Make sure that your medical practice has a leading-edge performance management system that adequately measures and tracks employee performance. Your medical practice should also have up-to-date policies on employee promotion and transfers.

Incentives and rewards programs help retain top talent and motivate employees to improve performance. Therefore, it is recommended that group practices develop policies about incentives and rewards programs for the staff.

Chapter 3 **Managing an Effective Staffing Strategy**

STAFFING A MEDICAL OFFICE requires a strong understanding of staff skills and abilities tied in with organizational goals. Staffing numbers and mix need to be tied into the organizational goals. The types of staff needed relates to the skill mix and knowledge that the practice requires. Hiring a registered nurse for a physician practice was a popular approach in the past. Currently, a medical practice will assess the skills needed for a practice and may decide that a medical assistant, rather than a nurse, can perform the skills needed for the practice. The goal may be to have the person room a patient, take vitals, learn the chief complaint, and handle minimal patient education. This staffing assessment helps the practice to determine the best mix of skills and abilities for which to recruit.

New Staff

The timing to bring on new staff is always a challenge. Sometimes staff members complain that they are overworked and need additional staff. That overworked perception may be specific to a particular day, due to understaffed departments as a result of vacations, or from additional tasks that have been assumed due to a special, time-specific project. It is critical for the medical practice executive to assess the needs of a department and determine under what circumstances and timing the staff may need more help.

Some organizations have a structure and culture that does not allow certain staffing changes to occur. A medical practice with an exclusive registered nursing staff is not as open to considering hiring medical assistants or licensed practical nurses as would be a medical practice that already has a mix of medical assistants and registered nurses. A culture that only has physicians may not be open to hiring nonphysician providers.

◾ Alternative Staffing

Nonphysician Providers

A nonphysician provider can include a nurse practitioner, physician assistant, or nurse midwife, among others. If hired, a nonphysician provider should function in a medical practice under the direction and supervision of a practicing, licensed physician. The supervising physician must have the appropriate training, experience, and competence to supervise the nonphysician provider. The physician practice should determine whether a nonphysician provider would fit within the group and determine the types of duties and functions that he or she would perform. Many arrangements have failed because of lack of preparation for a nonphysician provider and a clear definition of the roles and duties of that position in advance. Many practices have found that the consumer patient rates nonphysician providers very high due to their focus on patient education and the longer time that the nonphysician provider gives to the patient.

Nonphysician providers can be accepted in one physician specialty or region of the United States but not accepted in another specialty or region. The use of a nurse midwife in an OB/GYN practice is common, but a nonphysician provider may be less common in a region of the United States, where malpractice rates are high. Strategically, the medical practice executive should determine whether the use of a nonphysician provider would work from many perspectives, including economic, operational, and strategic.

Part-Time Employees

Part-time employees can help the medical practice address changing practice needs. A part-time employee may be able to work flexible hours based on the patient load or have the time to cover employees who are on vacation, sick, or being trained. A part-time employee may want to grow into a full-time position, but may want the flexibility of fewer hours now and more hours later.

Outsourcing

Staffing costs or restrictions may require a medical practice to outsource certain functions. Common outsourced functions may be information technology services, housekeeping, maintenance, coding, and billing. These functions, as outsourced services, have their own set of deliverables and expectations. Outsourcing may be able to achieve greater cost savings than if those services were performed in-house.

◼ Benchmarks

The number of staff needed can be tied into benchmarking data of like organizations. A new physician will not require two new staff members, and a pediatrician practicing at the 90th percentile of production may need more than two staff to support the practice. The number of staff should be based on productivity measures, hours of operation, skills required, available technology, and other resources within the group. For example, a practice that has an electronic health record and automated telephone response system in place may not need the same number of staff as a practice of the same size that has paper medical records and no telephone automation.

Full-time-equivalent (FTE) ratios provide a benchmark for the medical practice to follow. They may be guidelines or measures of productivity, production, and/or efficiency. For example, 4.5 FTEs per physician may be a good ratio for a physician achieving production at the 99th percentile, but a bad ratio for a physician at the 10th percentile. FTE ratios can help the medical practice guide staffing decisions and outcomes.

The Medical Group Management Association provides resources that benchmark physician-to-staff ratios based on numerous factors, such as physician specialty, medical ownership, and practice size. A busy family practice physician seeing 40 patients a day will require more staff than a busy urologist seeing 15 patients a day due to the volume of patients seen in a primary-care vs. specialty-care practice. In addition, the staff ratio needs to be broken down with respect to the types of people needed to ensure that the appropriate mix of staff skills is available to support the physician.

Planning work-force needs is both an art and a science. Staff ratios may meet benchmarked data, but they may still be ineffective if the staff members are not well trained and other resources of automation, coordination, and teamwork are not in place.

■ Changes in the Organization and Market

Jobs evolve over time, and new types of jobs may emerge. A medical practice needs to change with the times and be open to employment changes based on the needs of the practice. Twenty years ago, no one in a medical practice would have considered having either a chief information officer (CIO) in a medical practice or a telephone triage nurse. However, with the growth of information technology and automated applications, a CIO may be needed to handle the complexities and management of these applications. With the growth of managed care, requirements for preauthorizations for certain medical procedures and hospital admissions, and a more sophisticated and educated patient population, a telephone triage nurse can help address many of these new issues.

Expectations also change over time. A medical secretary hired to transcribe medical notes and answer the telephone for a physician may need to change job functions when "talk technology" eliminates the need for transcription and a call center is developed to answer the telephone. An employee who doesn't adapt well to change will become a liability instead of an asset when change is required within the practice.

Shortages in the labor pool create tremendous strain on the medical practice and may limit the practice's ability to meet current or growing patient needs. With a shortage of radiology technologists, a medical practice may not be able to expand hours of operation in the evenings or weekends. A strategy will help the medical group decide how aggressive it wants to be in recruiting hard-to-find staff.

■ Plans

Strategic and Business Plans

A strategic plan followed by a detailed business plan will help a medical practice to address its changing needs over time. A strategic plan is usually created for a three- to five-year period and articulates the practice's vision for the future. For example, the medical practice may have an aging medical group and need to recruit younger physicians. The vision of physician recruitment should be integrated into a business plan for the recruitment process. Planning for the future helps the medical group to become proactive and not reactive to a changing environment.

If a medical practice is open eight hours a day and five days a week, the space is used only 24 percent of the time. If a medical practice wants to expand its productivity, it can either see more patients every hour or expand its hours of operation. Developing a second medical office location for the practice can be an expensive endeavor unless the practice decides to pilot a new location through a time-share arrangement in which a physician shares space with another physician who already has an established practice.

Human resources may lead a strategic effort toward disseminated authority or may require decisions to be made by a board of directors or senior physician/administrative leader. Because the human resource department is a cost center, careful consideration is made on what the cost and benefits are for a particular decision.

Budget Plans

Eighty percent of a medical practice's budget may be focused on staffing. This creates huge challenges for the medical administrator to provide qualified, well-trained staff at a competitive price. A medical practice executive should consider how overtime, shift differential pay, and employee status (part time vs. full time) impact the bottom line in short- and long-term budgets.

■ Staffing and Scheduling

Staffing is both an art and a science. Developing an effective schedule based on staffing mix, hours needed, and skills performed will work if there are enough staff members to draw from. A mix of full-time, part-time, and as-needed staff who can work days, evenings, and weekends provide scheduling flexibility for the practice manager.

Schedules can vary based on physician or patient needs. Medical practices may vary employee shifts and hours based on employee preferences. For example, an employee may be attracted to three 12-hour shifts because it allows that employee to be off four days during the week, even though the employee has to work long hours for three days. In contrast, another employee may want only 8-hour shifts because of limitations in day care. Even though flexible schedules are logistically challenging, they can be strong employee satisfiers. Rotating employee shifts to work every third weekend may be preferable to required weekend shifts every week. These flexible schedule blocks can meet employee needs and meet the needs of the organization to provide staffing during nontraditional hours.

Chapter 4 **Developing and Implementing Staff Compensation and Benefit Plans**

◼ Basic Compensation

Compensation must be fair, equitable, and related to the job tasks that the person is expected to perform. An employee may initially be paid based on his or her skill, knowledge, or competency-based expertise. The higher the employee's skill or competency, the higher his or her pay. For example, a manager with a bachelor's degree is usually paid less than someone with a master's degree.

If an incentive program is developed, it should be fair, consistent, and measurable. The criteria should easily be understood and be able to be tracked. A performance-based compensation model is the most common type of compensation model provided to employees. It is based on merit and is easy to develop, track, and administer. An employee is hired at a salaried or hourly wage and provided wage increases based on how well he or she performed in a previous period. Incentive pay options allow the employee to receive a bonus based on completing predetermined job goals. If the goals aren't achieved, the employee doesn't receive an increase in pay. For example, a medical group may decide that an average performer receives a 3 percent increase and an exceptional performer receives a 4 percent increase. A determination of the difference between average and high performers is needed for such merit increases.

Physician Compensation

A way in which a medical practice compensates its physicians for services provided is one of the most important issues affecting a medical group, and can ultimately determine the success or failure of the practice. A physician may be paid based on knowledge or skill. A physician with dual-board certification may be paid more than a physician without that certification. A cardiologist may be paid more than a pediatrician, based on the cardiologist's skill, job knowledge, and additional years of training. In addition, a physician may be provided with a fixed salary based on anticipated work with a formula for a bonus or incentive if the workload is exceeded.

Physician compensation will reflect a medical practice's mix of physicians and its legal and cost structure, along with its culture, history, and external influences. Regardless of the plan, the compensation method must reflect the medical practice's goals. It must reward productivity that is consistent with the mission and values of the organization. It must be fair and consistently administered, simple and easily understood, and comply with the law. It should be aligned with the financial needs of the organization and allow the medical group to retain current providers and recruit new providers. Above all, the plan must be fair.[17]

Staff Compensation

The medical practice executive should routinely evaluate position compensation based on internal and external factors, evaluating the initial pay offered an employee and the merit increases that an employee receives over time. Adjustments in pay tables and ranges should occur at the same time each year to allow for a consistent process and approach unless there are some extenuating circumstances. Pay adjustments should be communicated to employees in writing, including the reason for the adjustment. A poorly run program may allow inconsistencies to enter a system, thus creating unintentional pay inequities.

The marketplace needs to be considered when developing compensation scales. The marketplace must always be considered in recruiting well-qualified employees and to keep employee turnover low. In addition, an economic condition, such as a period of inflation or recession, will impact the kinds of pay scales that are offered to employees.

The local market may require a medical practice to take a different approach from national or regional approaches. A medical practice located in a rural or urban area may need to offer a higher rate of pay or other incentives to encourage a person to join the practice. A potential employee needs to see that the higher compensation or benefits are worth the potential change in quality of life.

A practice may need to recruit outside of its local area due to shortages in a certain type of position. A tougher labor market to recruit a particular position will result in a medical group having to pay a higher market rate for that position. For example, a pharmacist shortage may require the medical practice to seek candidates from nearby metropolitan areas or even pursue a national search. These commitments become very expensive recruiting efforts and require additional recruiting support to deal with new issues of travel costs, introduction to the community, costs of a real estate agent, housing relocation expenses, and other transition costs.

The medical practice executive should evaluate pay scales periodically to ensure that there is parity within the pay grades. Sometimes a position within the marketplace changes and requires a modification of pay. When new hires are brought into the organization at a higher rate of pay than is traditional, internal parity needs to be made for other comparable positions within the organization to ensure equitable pay.

Job-Driven Compensation

How compensation scales are developed determines how successful the medical group is in attracting and retaining employees. Difficult-to-recruit positions, such as certified coders and nuclear medicine technologists, may have special or higher pay scales. Some positions may require a higher-than-average starting salary to be competitive in the marketplace.

Some positions are difficult to recruit because of intense external competitiveness. There may be a shortage of qualified candidates for a certain position in the local market due to few if any formal training programs or an increase in need due to a growing industry. For example, nurses are difficult to recruit because there are so many groups trying to recruit the same labor pool – from hospitals, nursing homes, and home care agencies, to schools, medical groups, and public health agencies. This external competitiveness will lead organizations to consider paying nurses at higher rates or deciding to run a practice with staff that has lower skills levels (e.g., medical assistants).

Certain positions may even warrant a medical practice to offer a sign-on bonus for difficult-to-fill positions. With shortages in nurses, radiology technologists, professional coders, and other competitive positions, other options may be retention bonuses given to the employee after staying on the job for a 6- or 12-month period.

Recruitment packages need to be sensitive to the current work force and current staffing. If co-workers see that tremendous resources are placed on recruiting additional staff but no resources are devoted to retain current employees, there may be perceived inequity issues, which may prompt certain employees to leave the medical practice and thus create a larger recruitment issue for the practice.

In addition, wage compression can occur wherein all the positions in a like category make similar wages because of the labor market. For example, all professional coders may make a similar wage regardless of experience because most of the coders are being paid toward the top of the compensation range. This compression makes it difficult to manage ongoing resources for other employees who may expect the same type of plan for themselves.

Pay Grades/Steps

Published salary surveys use data from internal and external sources to develop a tool that can be invaluable to a medical group to know the financial factors to consider regarding employee compensation. Such tools include salary groups and pay scales within each salary group. Professional associations such as the Medical Group

Management Association (MGMA) print benchmarked salary data for physicians and staff. In addition, the federal government publishes national data on certain positions that can help a medical practice determine the kind of pay scale it wants to have for a particular position. These updated data help the medical practice executive determine whether the practice's ranges need to be adjusted to reflect changing market rates.

Salary survey data in addition to job structure within the organization are used to develop pay grades and ranges for positions within the medical group. Salary grades group similar jobs together with the same pay grade and pay rate. The number of salary grades is determined by the medical group based on the types and number of positions within the practice. Salary grades have a minimum, midpoint, and maximum for each pay grade and have some overlap among other pay grades to allow for differences in employee experience levels in different ranges. For example, a newly hired employee in pay grade 24 may make less than a highly experienced employee in pay grade 23. A compensation strategy that develops fewer and broader pay grades simplifies pay grade structure and allows employees to achieve higher pay in the same range.

The development of salary-increase guides helps to establish clear expectations and allows for better budgeting. If a practice usually has half of the employees receiving a 3 percent increase and half receiving a 4 percent increase, then the administrator can budget the maximum amount of money that will be allocated to salary increases for the next fiscal year.

Pay grades can have a maximum pay scale so that an employee may hit the top of the range. Organizations need to determine whether the person is "redlined" so that he or she is not eligible for any pay increases or whether there is a special incentive program available to senior employees.

Informal Salary Information Sources

Informal salary surveys allow the organization to respond to changing market forces. During the recruitment process, HR professionals glean large amounts of information from candidates, including salary and benefits data. If potential candidates will not work for a medical group because of "low pay," this kind of information should be revealed during the interview process. Also, new hires may validate the competitive pay and benefits of the employer when they sign up for their benefits in the new organization. Data from these types of encounters can be invaluable for the organization.

In addition, peers can share data about why employees are leaving a certain organization, and exit interviews can provide other anecdotal information about an employee's personal experience. For example, an employee may share that he is leaving the medical group to work at a competitor's organization in the same job for a one-dollar-an-hour increase in pay. However, all the factors would need to be considered. In this case, at the competitor's office, the employee would receive an additional $2,080 in annual salary ($1 × 2,080 full-time hours worked per year), but he would also have to pay $3,000 out-of-pocket for benefits. The net effect would be a salary loss of $920 due to increased benefits costs. This result suggests that the employee might have additional or unstated reasons for leaving the organization.

Confidentiality of Compensation Data

The medical group needs to determine what types of compensation/ pay information can be shared with employees and what information should remain private. For example, a group may elect to keep salaries private, but communicate the bonus structure with everyone, telling staff and physicians that is was calculated based on seniority, pay grade, or other factors. Private information is, obviously, private and confidential. It should not be shared with other people and should remain protected information in the employee file.

A medical practice should have a policy on what type of pay information is shared. A closed policy is one that does not openly share pay grades or ranges. For example, a position is posted and the pay grade is 23, which means that the position's minimum pay is $12 per hour and maximum pay is $16 per hour. This open policy allows the employee to know whether he or she is interested in this position or not. A closed policy would not post a pay grade, may not openly share that information, and would share pay information only to a final candidate being considered. Knowing whether to share certain kinds of pay information helps the medical practice executive to focus on following its policies.

Sharing such data can create conflict and tension. However, certain groups, such as government agencies, share salary information openly, and this is a common expectation for this group. Overall, salary information should be kept confidential and staff should be encouraged to maintain confidentiality regarding salaries.

◢ Formal Benefits

Whereas an employee's direct pay is easily seen, the indirect pay, consisting of the employee's benefits, retirement benefits, and social security, is often overlooked. Formal benefits may include medical, dental, and vision plans, short- and long-term disability insurance, life insurance, pension plan, savings and investment plans, unemployment insurance, and workers' compensation premiums, among others. These benefits usually have a shared cost between the employer and employee based on a certain percentage. In larger organizations, the pay/benefit mix in total compensation could be 20 percent of the employee's wages. For example, an employee making $30,000 per year could expect to receive approximately $6,000 in additional benefits from the organization.

A flexible benefit plan allows the employee to choose from a range of benefits that best meet his or her current needs. There may be a dollar-amount cap to apply to those benefits. For example, one employee may have a $1,500 cap that is applied to a $1,000 medical premium and a $500 vision premium, and another employee may apply his or her $1,500 to a $750 dental premium and $750 toward a medical premium.

Benchmarking data helps the employer determine whether the benefit package being offered to employees is competitive within the marketplace. If the market shows that employers generally provide benefits up to 20 percent of the employee payroll and a particular employer provides only 10 percent, that factor may influence whether an employee will join the organization.

Benefits have short- and long-term effects on the employee base. A practice may decide to fund a certain benefit today but regret its financial impact on the group in the future. As an example, in the past, the automobile industry decided to fully fund retiree health premiums when costs were well within control and there were few retirees. However, with an aging work force and retirees living longer, the financial impact has become cost prohibitive, prompting the industry to decide how to handle benefits for the future. These lessons learned can help medical groups design benefit packages that are fair, equitable, and affordable for both the employee and employer.

Goal-Driven Benefits

Equity Ownership

Equity ownership may allow a physician to participate in owning a part of the medical practice, which would allow the physician to participate in any financial gains. In for-profit organizations that allow stock to be purchased, an employee can purchase stock in the company and have equity ownership. On the downside, equity ownership also means sharing losses.

Some medical groups have shareholders and nonshareholders. Compensation methods will be different for the two groups. For example, depending on the legal structure, a physician may have stock options or direct ownership in a medical group. This arrangement will impact how the physician is paid.

Profit Sharing

A medical group may decide to offer its employees the opportunity to participate in a profit-sharing program that provides employees with additional pay if the medical group meets or exceeds its financial goals. The challenge is to decide how much of the profit will be distributed and to whom. Or, bonuses may be provided if the practice meets its financial goals.

As an incentive to achieve department goals, a medical practice may decide to provide a team reward if the team achieves a certain financial outcome. For example, a medical group with an urgent care center may provide an incentive for the team who sees more than 50 patients a day. This goal would mean the team would be required to get all the patients through the center on a timely basis and avoid any walk-outs from the clinic due to timeliness issues.

Gainsharing

Gainsharing is a process by which employees are involved in performance enhancements and share the financial benefits of these improvements made by the medical practice. Gainsharing is a common practice among Fortune 500 companies. Unlike bonuses that are provided annually, gainsharing allows regular financial payments to be made to the employee, such as on a monthly or quarterly basis. The system instills immediate understanding by the employee on what is needed to be accomplished to achieve a gainsharing bonus. Although the system may be incomplete on providing incentives to employees to achieve all organizational goals, this tool has been used for many companies to achieve phenomenal results.

Insurance Benefits

The types of insurance that may be offered usually apply to health or life.

Health Insurance

With more than 40 million people in the United States currently lacking health insurance,[18] and many Americans believing health care is a basic right, access to health insurance coverage is a key benefit for a medical practice. Employees may seek employment based on whether the employer offers health insurance. It is common for smaller medical practices not to offer health insurance to their employees, but most larger practices have to offer health insurance to competitively recruit employees.

Some medical groups contract with external groups to handle their health insurance coverage. Other medical practices may cover their own health insurance through a self-insured plan. Regardless of the arrangement, health insurance must be managed effectively and efficiently, with cost containment being one of the largest issues plaguing medical practices today.

In addition to basic health insurance, additional specific health-related insurance may include the following:

- *Dental, vision, and hearing insurance.* Dental and/or vision insurance offerings can be employer and/or employee funded and offer coverage under health maintenance organization, preferred provider organization, or traditional plans. Hearing and vision insurance may be options for those employees and/or dependents who experience hearing and/or vision problems.

- *In-house medical services.* As an employee benefit, medical practices may offer access to certain types of medical services within the organization. Services may range from free access to physician services to reduced fees for pharmaceuticals and medical supplies.

- *Travel insurance.* For medical practices that require employees to travel to different locations for business, offering travel insurance in case of problems is a common, and inexpensive, benefit.

- *Long-term and short-term disability insurance.* Short-term disability coverage defines plan days covered, plan funding, and what is and is not considered a short-term disability. Plans that allow pregnancy as a short-term disability are very popular for employers with a potentially child-bearing work force.

- *Postretirement medical benefits.* With continued concerns about access to health insurance, some medical groups offer employees access to medical benefits after retirement. Whereas access to medical benefits through the Consolidated Omnibus Budget Reconciliation Act of 1985 (COBRA) are offered for up to 18 months after an employee leaves an organization, postretirement medical benefits are offered only to those employees who officially retire. Qualified retirees may need to meet certain age requirements, and payment of medical benefits may be based on years of service at the organization prior to retiring.

- *Long-term care plans.* As the population continues to age, long-term care plans are becoming more popular. For an employee/employer contribution, the plan covers the cost for a certain percentage of care provided in an approved long-term-care facility.

Life Insurance

Life insurance may be just for the employee, or the practice may offer a plan for the employee and dependents. The plan will have limits usually based on the employee's income or a percentage of his or her income. In addition to life insurance policies that cover general death benefits, some employers offer an additional coverage for accidental death, such as due to automobile accident, plane crash, or similar accident.

Retirement and Severance Benefits

Pension Plans

Pension plans allow the employee to have money available for retirement. The pension plan may be fully funded by the employer or may have joint employer and employee contributions.

Severance Pay

As more organizations are downsizing, going bankrupt, or going through mergers, acquisitions, and consolidations, they have developed a severance pay policy for employees whose positions are eliminated. Usually, these policies are based on the employees' employment status (full- vs. part-time), the employee's class (exempt vs. nonexempt, management vs. executive), and years of service (less than one year, one to five years, five or more years). These differentiations will determine the level of severance provided to an employee.

■ Issues Related to Benefits

Benefit Cost Sharing

Employers determine which benefits are employer-paid, which are employee-paid, and which are shared by both the employer and employee. Inflation, malpractice premium increases, and reduced reimbursement from managed care plans, among other factors, are affecting the bottom line of many practices. Therefore, the employee is picking up more of the cost of benefits. The employer must be careful with this strategy, though, because it may lead to higher turnover and a medical practice that is less effective in the marketplace. Although this shift in payment responsibility may be a cost-effective approach for the employer, it may strap the employee with higher costs and a perceived drop in quality of life, leading to employee dissatisfaction.

A medical practice may choose to be self-funding for a certain part of its benefit costs. For example, it may contract out its life insurance and short-term disability benefits but self-fund its health insurance costs through its own insurance plan or medical malpractice through an offshore captive insurance company.

Eligibility

Benefit plans can be established for certain employee types and classes of employees. A medical practice can define the difference between full-time and part-time employment for benefit purposes. A full-time position may be 36+ hours of work per week, which allows the employee to participate in the full-time benefit plan, whereas part-time benefits would be available for employees working from 20 to 35 hours a week. Those employees who work less than 20 hours each week could be considered ineligible for benefits. More benefits would be available for the full-time employee as an incentive to work full time. Examples would be that a full-time employee would receive reduced premiums on health insurance and an employer-paid short-term disability benefit, whereas a part-time employee would receive a higher medical premium and no short-term disability benefit.

Benefits could also vary based on job class so that the physician receives a different type of benefit structure than the staff. The benefit package, however, needs to be carefully designed with appropriate human resources and legal counsel to ensure that the plan meets federal and state legal requirements and doesn't violate any specific laws. For example, the medical practice may want to offer a pension plan to physicians and employees but offer a shorter vesting period for physicians. That change in benefit may not be allowed based on how the practice and employees are organized. Legal counsel can review pension laws to determine what kinds of variables are allowed.

Legal and Tax Issues

Retirement plans can be qualified or nonqualified. Qualified plans do not discriminate among employees, are tax-exempt, and offer a tax deferral benefit for employee and employer contributions. Qualified plans allow the medical practice a tax deduction for plan contributions wherein employees do not pay taxes on plan assets until they are distributed, and plan earnings are tax deferred. To maintain a qualified status, an employer must follow the requirements of the Internal Revenue Service (IRS), the Department of Labor (DOL), and the Employee Retirement Income Security Act of 1974 (ERISA).

A nonqualified plan has easy plan adoption and no coverage, eligibility, or participation requirements. It allows contributions beyond caps established for qualified plans. A medical practice can decide to provide nonqualified deferred compensation plans to only a select group of employees (e.g., physicians). Whereas a qualified plan must be written and must meet participation, vesting, and funding requirements, a nonqualified plan need not meet these requirements. A nonqualified plan allows the employee to get more compensation.

However, nonqualified plans have drawbacks. The medical practice won't claim a tax deduction for employee amounts until the employee receives that money as income, perhaps many years in the future. The employee may not receive the money at all, however, if the medical practice becomes insolvent, because that money is subject to the claims of the medical practice's creditors; in other words, it is unsecured.

Some benefits are legally required, such as payment of unemployment benefits, workers' compensation premiums, and taking out monies for federal, state, and local taxes. When designing a compensation and benefits program, the medical practice must be aware of the following laws and how they may impact the development of the plan.

ERISA

For the medical practice, ERISA is a federal law that sets minimum standards for voluntary established pension and health plans to protect plan participants. ERISA requires participants to be provided with information such as plan features and funding, participation standards, vesting, benefit accrual and funding, fiduciary responsibilities for assets, and a grievance and appeals process.

HIPAA

The Health Insurance Portability and Accountability Act of 1996 (HIPAA) was approved to amend the Internal Revenue Code of 1986. Its primary purpose is to improve portability and continuity of health insurance coverage, eliminate misuse in health insurance and its delivery, promote medical savings account use, improve access to long-term-care services, and simplify health insurance administration.

COBRA

COBRA amends ERISA, the Internal Revenue Code, and the Public Health Service Act to ensure the continuation of group health coverage that otherwise would have been terminated. It allows certain former employees and dependents to temporarily continue health coverage at group rates, which are usually less expensive than private health coverage. In general, the law applies to health plans with 20+ employees and requires that the plan have rules detailing how an individual becomes entitled to these benefits. Life insurance is not covered under COBRA.

Medical Practice Payroll Obligations

Every medical practice, as an employer, must report to the IRS with regard to the income paid to each employee. The medical practice should determine the amount of income tax to withhold. The medical practice, based on its size, will either deposit the taxes it withholds for future payment to the IRS, or will send it directly to the IRS. The three components of federal payroll taxes are federal income taxes withheld from the employee's wages, the employees' share of Federal Insurance Contributions Act (FICA) taxes, and the employer's matching share of FICA taxes.

FICA comprises a Medicare hospital insurance tax of 1.45 percent on all taxable wages and Old-Age, Survivors, and Disability Insurance (OASDI) of 6.2 percent (commonly called Social Security). Therefore, a medical practice must withhold 7.65 percent of each employee's wage and match this amount with its own funds.

In addition to these taxes, the medical practice may be liable to pay IRS Code Section 457 plans, workers' compensation insurance, and/or unemployment insurance.

Social Security

The Social Security Act is the law governing most operations of the Social Security program. The original Social Security Act was enacted in 1935 and subsequent amendments comprise 20 titles. The OASDI program is authorized by Title II of the Social Security Act. Social Security is usually referred to as a "tax." It is actually the amount of contribution based on a percent of earnings, up to an annual maximum, that must be paid by employers and employees on wages from employment under FICA. Usually, medical practices withhold contributions from wages, add an equal amount of contributions, and pay both on a current basis.

IRS Code Section 457/Deferred Compensation

Section 457 plans are nonqualified, deferred compensation plans established by state or local government and tax-exempt employers. If a medical practice is considered to be a tax-exempt employer, it would qualify to provide this type of plan. The practice could establish either eligible or ineligible plans, which are subject to the specific requirements and deferral limitations of Section 457 of the IRS code.

Workers' Compensation

The concept of workers' compensation (generally known as "workers' comp") dates back 100 years, to 1908, when it was enacted for federal employees. It relates to the liability of the employer to pay damages for employee injuries incurred while the employee is on the job. Workers' compensation includes an elective schedule of compensation and provides a procedure to determine liability and compensation. It is actually an insurance program that pays an employee for medical and disability benefits for work-related injuries or certain diseases. If an employee is injured on the job, the employee's medical treatment costs are paid by the workers' compensation policy. If the employee has a job-related injury that prevents him or her from working, the employee will receive weekly income through the policy until able to return to work. Medical practices must either obtain coverage by purchasing a workers' compensation insurance policy or become licensed to "self-insure" by the state labor commissioner.

Unemployment Insurance

Unemployment compensation was created by the Social Security Act of 1935 to help eligible people who, through no fault of their own, are unemployed. Monetary benefits are usually determined according to the amount of former wages and/or weeks of work. The program is funded by employer taxes, either federal or state, and is a partnership between the federal and state governments wherein the program is based on federal law but administered by state employees under state law. Each state creates its own program within the guidelines of the federal government. The state statute develops the eligibility and disqualification provisions, benefit amount, state tax base, and state rate.

▪ Other Benefits

Recruiting Bonuses

Employees may be provided with a "recruitment bonus" or "referral bonus" if a person is referred to the medical practice, accepts the position, and stays in the position for a certain period of time. This bonus generates employee buy-in of the recruitment process, creates awareness of difficult-to-recruit positions, and encourages employees to network with others to promote the organization for future employment.

Paid Time Off

An employee may be afforded time off if it does not conflict with the needs of the department and is pre-approved by a supervisor. Moreover, employers are currently moving to a flexible program of paid time off (PTO) that combines time off for sick leave, vacation, holidays, and jury duty into one pool. In this way, the employee manages one "bucket" of time instead of having different buckets of time. The PTO plan mitigates situations in which employees would dip into an unrelated bucket, such as an employee with a sick child who inappropriately draws on the "sick time" bucket because there is no time left in his or her vacation time bucket.

Financial Planning/Counseling

While medical practices may provide retirement resources for the employee through Social Security and a pension plan, those resources may not be enough for the employee at the time of retirement to maintain a certain quality of life. As a result, a voluntary investment plan such as a 401(k) plan would allow the employee to defer receiving compensation in order to have the amount contributed to the plan for future use at retirement. Information on employee assistance programs (EAPs), including financial counseling, can be found in Chapter 2.

Housing Finance Assistance

Owning a house is an integral part of the "American dream," and organizations can help employees achieve that dream through offering housing finance assistance. An employee can benefit from housing finance assistance, including financial planning, exploration of options available, and reduced rates through group consortiums.

Child Care/Elder Care

Caring for family, such as children or elderly parents, is an important employee value. A medical practice that helps employees address these issues can be a strong employee satisfier. A medical practice may choose to offer a plan for the employee to save money pre-tax to pay for these services or may actually offer these services through the practice at a reduced employee rate.

Charitable Matching Contributions

Some medical practices offer a charitable matching program that matches a certain percentage of funds that an employee contributes to a charity. For example, if an employee contributes $100 to the American Red Cross, the employer might contribute 50 percent of the employee's contribution, or $50, to that agency, too. Certain limitations may apply to this benefit, such as contribution caps and select charities.

Individual Retirement Accounts

An Individual Retirement Account (IRA) allows an employee to invest pre-tax dollars in an investment plan that is managed by the employee. It is a self-directed, employee-funded retirement plan. Employers may choose to contribute money to this type of plan instead of managing their own pension plan.

Informal Benefits

Informal benefits, such as gift certificates, lunches out, or other tokens of appreciation, are discussed in Chapter 2.

Retirement Planning

Much has been written about the generational diversity in today's work force – particularly contrasting the Baby Boomer generation and Generation X. Unfortunately, neither group is saving at a sufficient rate to provide for its retirement. A recent study by the Center for Retirement Research at Boston College concluded that 44 percent of households with working-age adults, including 49 percent of Generation Xers (born between 1965 and 1982), 44 percent of late Boomers (born between 1955 and 1964), and 35 percent of early Boomers (born between 1946 and 1954), are at risk for lacking sufficient funds to maintain the working adults' standard of living in retirement. These statistics assume the adults work until age 65 and annuitize all their financial assets, and include receipts from reverse mortgages.[19]

A qualified retirement plan benefits medical practice owners and employees by providing a mechanism for accumulating retirement savings. It also provides significant tax benefits to the practice and its employees, a competitive advantage to the practice for attracting and retaining good employees.

Physician Retirement Savings and Wealth Accumulation

According to Thomas J. Stanley, PhD, and William D. Danko, PhD, authors of *The Millionaire Next Door,* physicians have a low propensity to accumulate substantial personal wealth compared to individuals in other high-earning occupations. The authors attribute this problem, in part, to physicians' late start beginning their practices after many years of education and professional training. The substantial debt obtained to finance this education also hinders a physician's ability to save. Finally, because physicians typically spend long hours taking care of their patients' physical health, they often have little time to devote to managing their own financial health.[20] Because retirement plan assets often comprise a significant portion of a physician's personal savings, selecting and managing these plans is crucial, not just to the practice but also as a part of the physician-owners' overall financial plan.

◼ Tax Advantages

The first tax benefit offered by qualified retirement plans and simplified employee pension (SEP) plans is that contributions to the plans are fully tax-deductible when made in accordance with tax laws. This means that neither the practice (its owners in the case of a pass-through entity) nor its employees pay current income taxes on the employer contributions. Second, if an employer permits employee deferrals under a 401(k) arrangement, those contributions are not currently subject to income taxes, although these amounts are subject to applicable Medicare and Social Security taxes for both the employee and the employer.

Another important tax benefit, especially for plan participants, is that the earnings on qualified retirement plan contributions are not subject to income taxes until they are withdrawn from the plan. This allows plan assets to grow and compound at a significantly faster rate than investments in a taxable account.

As discussed later in this chapter, distributions from the plan are generally subject to income taxes. But, if funds have accumulated in the plan for many years, the absence of income taxes increases the potential for wealth accumulation for the physician-owners and their long-term employees. As discussed earlier, an overlooked but extremely important aspect of retirement plans is the inability to access the funds until retirement. This results in a forced savings program for the physician and typically allows them to retire with a comfortable standard of living.

Attracting and Retaining Quality Staff Members

Many speculate that the upcoming retirement of members of the large Baby Boomer generation will contribute to a future shortage of qualified employees. Because of the technical nature of the skills required in health care and the anticipated increase in the demand for health care, predictions indicate that the health care industry will be especially hard hit by the shortage. Indeed, shortages are currently evident in nursing and laboratory positions.

According to a study by Hewitt, 93 percent of Generation X and 92 percent of Generation Y expect their 401(k) plans to provide income for retirement.[21] Yet, 2006 DOL statistics indicate that only 43 percent of workers employed by private businesses in the United States participate in defined contribution retirement plans (401(k) plans) and only 20 percent participate in defined benefit plans.[22] Having a qualified retirement plan makes an employer more attractive to potential employees and helps them retain existing employees, thus giving the practice a competitive advantage in the war for talent. Most practices currently offer a qualified plan, so to remain competitive, usually employers must have one.

◼ Importance of Management and Compliance

Qualified retirement plans are subject to a number of federal laws and regulations promulgated by both the DOL and IRS – penalties for noncompliance can be significant. The trustees and employer sponsor of a plan must ensure proper handling of internal administrative matters, such as remitting deferrals and employer funding on a timely basis. These administrative functions are often delegated to the practice administrator to oversee. The assistance of an outside third-party administrator is an excellent resource to the practice administrator in this role.

Because the plan's financial assets, which are often significant, are important to the retirement security of the practice's employees and physician-owners, the trustees of the plan (often the physicians) should perform due diligence to ensure that the plan assets are effectively managed. The DOL requires that plan assets be diversified and prudently managed to minimize the potential for large losses.[23] Using third-party vendors to assist in the investment selection, ongoing communication, and staff education achieves this diversification.

An administrator should develop the knowledge and skills necessary to facilitate selection of the practice's qualified retirement plan and its administration and regulatory compliance. This chapter provides a basic overview of some of the significant issues common to a medical practice's qualified retirement plan.

▰ Types of Plans

Practices will ordinarily choose from several popular options in retirement plans. Because practices usually rely on one or more outside advisors in connection with selecting, maintaining, and administering a plan, the practice administrator does not generally need to be aware of all the technical aspects of the plan. A general knowledge of the various options is sufficient to assist the administrator in assuring physicians and other leaders that the group has considered the available plan designs.

Defined Benefit Plans

A defined benefit plan is one in which the employer contributes an amount necessary to ensure a fixed level of benefits to the employees when they retire. These plans are more complex than defined contribution plans. They require the services of an enrolled actuary to compute the required contribution. Contributions to these plans are mandatory; if a practice fails to meet the minimum funding standards, it can be subject to excise taxes. Furthermore, the practice may need to purchase insurance coverage to guarantee the benefits from the Pension Benefit Guaranty Corporation (PBGC).[24]

The use of defined benefit plans by employers has decreased significantly over the past few decades. In 1983, 60 percent of households with a pension were covered by a defined benefit plan. This percentage dropped to 37 percent in 2006.[25] These plans are rarely found in the health care industry.

More recently, defined benefit plans have received increased attention from small employers. This has occurred because, at least in part, aging Baby Boomers realize that they have not saved enough for retirement and feel a degree of skepticism about the Social Security system.[26] Because defined benefit plans allow larger contributions for older employees, they may be appropriate for practices with older physicians who want to put away more money for retirement than the limitation imposed on defined contribution plans.[27] These plans might be prohibitively expensive for practices with a large number of older rank-and-file employees.

Defined Contribution Plans

While contributions to defined benefit plans are based on achieving a specific benefit, benefits available under a defined contribution plan are based on the contributions made to the plan by the employer, the employee, and the associated earnings on these contributions. An individual account is maintained for each participant, and that participant's benefit is based on the amount contributed to his or her account, plus any income, expenses, gains, losses, or forfeitures from other participants that are allocated to that account. This type of plan is relatively simple to administer and occurs often in medical practices.

Popular types of defined contribution plans include money purchase pension plans, profit-sharing plans (including 401(k) deferral features, integration or cross-tested), and 403(b) plans.

Money Purchase Pension Plans

A money purchase pension plan is a defined contribution plan in which the contributions are calculated in accordance with a formula, but the benefits are not guaranteed. Although these plans were once prevalent in medical practices, they have become less common because the annual funding is mandatory by the employer and, as a result, they offer less flexibility.

Profit-Sharing Plans

A profit-sharing plan often offers the most flexibility of all qualified retirement plans. The practice can elect to contribute as much as 25 percent of the annual covered compensation of all eligible employees. The maximum contribution on behalf of each employee and the amount of annual compensation considered for funding requirements increases periodically based on cost-of-living indexes. Although the employer is not required to make a contribution in any particular year, the IRS does require that contributions be more than sporadic. Revenue Ruling 80-146 states that if a profit-sharing plan receives no contributions for five consecutive years, the IRS will consider that plan to be terminated.[28] These plans are popular with medical practices.

401(k) Plans

Although frequently referred to as "plans" by many, including the media and even the IRS, 401(k) actually refers to an Internal Revenue Code section that describes a feature that can be added to either a profit-sharing or stock bonus plan. A 401(k) deferral allows participants to defer part of their pre-tax wages into the retirement plan. The plan might also include a provision in which the employer makes a matching contribution based on the employee's deferrals. The matching contribution is the only contingent benefit an employer may use to entice an employee to make elective deferrals to the 401(k) plan. Most businesses, including corporations, partnerships, sole proprietorships, limited liability entities, and nongovernmental tax-exempt organizations, may establish a 401(k) plan.[29]

Adding the 401(k) feature to a profit-sharing plan is popular with medical practices. Subject to the provisions discussed later in this chapter, this plan design allows for significant contributions for the physician-owners. It also provides the employee with the ability to provide for their own retirement, but often at a lower cost to the practice than other types of plans. Special catch-up deferral provisions are also available to plan participants who have attained at least age 50 during the plan year.

Safe Harbor 401(k) Plans

The basic principle of a safe harbor 401(k) plan is that the employer provides a certain minimum contribution in exchange for being able to eliminate deferral and matching nondiscrimination testing (discussed later in this chapter). The benefit of eliminating this testing is that employees with higher salaries can defer up to the annual limit (adjusted each year) without concern for what other employees defer.

Plan sponsors may choose between two types of contributions: a safe harbor nonelective contribution or a safe harbor matching contribution. These contributions must be 100-percent vested and are not available for hardship or other in-service withdrawals before age 59½. No minimum hours of service can be required and a participant cannot be required to be employed on the last day of the plan year. The nonelective contribution requires the employer to contribute 3 percent of each eligible employee's compensation for the year. The matching contribution requires the employer to match elective deferrals at the rate of 100 percent for the first 3 percent of compensation deferred, plus 50 percent of the next 2 percent deferred.

Plans that meet the safe harbor requirements are generally exempt from the top-heavy rules (discussed later in this chapter).

In addition, recent legislation allows plan sponsors to add a Roth provision to their 401(k) plan. This allows participants to make after-tax contributions to a plan. Subject to some special rules, this makes the future distributions of these contributions and their earnings tax-free.

Section 403(b) Plans

Also referred to as tax-sheltered annuities, Section 403(b) plans are retirement plans for employees of tax-exempt organizations, public schools, and cooperative hospital service organizations, as well as certain ministers. Physicians and other employees of universities and hospital systems might be eligible to participate in these plans. Like the 401(k) feature, these plans provide for elective deferrals under a salary reduction arrangement.[30]

Other Plans

Other plan options available include the SEP and cash balance plans.

Simplified Employee Pension Plans

A SEP plan is a not a qualified retirement plan; it is a type of IRA that is funded by the employer. It may receive annual contributions similar to those for money purchase pension and profit-sharing plans. The fact that these plans have fewer administrative requirements appeals to smaller practices; a major disadvantage, however, is that they do not receive protection from creditor claims because they are not qualified retirement plans.[31] Another disadvantage is that the funding immediately vests with the employee and they may withdraw the funds at any time after they are placed into the account.

This often results in adverse tax consequences to employees and negatively affects their long-term future.

Cash Balance Plans

Although a cash balance plan is technically a defined benefit plan, it performs like a hybrid arrangement with attributes of both a defined benefit and a defined contribution plan. One advantage to this arrangement is that it can provide for tax-deductible contributions in excess of the defined contribution limitations and can be designed to provide better parity in the level of benefits paid to older and younger workers than a traditional defined benefit plan.[32] An advanced technique often applied for physicians desiring to increase funding levels or to "catch up" on their funding shortfalls from prior years is to combine 401(k) profit-sharing and cash balance plans to achieve their objectives. Like other defined benefit plans, cash balance plans require actuarial services and are generally more expensive to administer than other defined contribution plans.

Setting Up the Plan

Once a practice has determined what type of plan best suits its needs, it must make decisions on how to design its plan.

Prototype vs. Individually Designed Plans

First, a practice must decide whether to adopt a *prototype plan* or have a plan designed specifically for the practice. Many investment vendors offer prototype plans, inexpensive "off-the-shelf" plan documents, to their clients. One potential disadvantage is that these plans may have limited design flexibility. For example, the practice is usually required to invest its plan assets with the plan's vendor, thus limiting investment flexibility.

Alternatively, a practice may have a professional, often an attorney, draft a plan specifically designed for its practice. Although individually designed plans are generally more flexible, they usually are more expensive to adopt and maintain, especially if future amendments are necessary.

Two key considerations are: (1) the expertise of the vendor providing the document, and (2) the operational and procedural components of the document. The plan document controls all aspects of the plan and should be reviewed by a professional familiar with qualified retirement plans.

Trustees and Fiduciaries

A trustee has a fiduciary responsibility to ensure that the retirement plan operates to secure the plan assets and to pay benefits and plan expenses for the sole benefit of the participants and beneficiaries. As fiduciaries, they have discretionary authority or control over the plan's operations, administration, and investments in accordance with the provisions of the plan document. Trustees must ensure that the plan complies with all regulations of the DOL and IRS.

The trustees may be officers of the group appointed by the board of directors or a professional trustee service offered by a third party. Although the trustees, such as officers of the practice, have the legal responsibility for plan operations, they typically use the services of outside advisors, including third-party administrators, employee benefit firms, accounting firms, and investment advisors. If a third party exercises discretionary powers over the plan investments, such as in the case of a registered investment advisor, that party may also be considered a fiduciary. Although attorneys, accountants, actuaries, insurance agents, and consultants frequently provide services in connection with a retirement plan, they are not considered fiduciaries unless they exercise discretionary authority over the plan or its assets.[33]

Plan Investments

The practice must make decisions on how it will handle plan investments. One decision is whether to have a *self-directed plan,* in which participants in defined contribution plans make their own investment decisions regarding their plan assets, or a *trustee-directed plan,* in which investment decisions are made by the trustees of the plan.

As previously discussed, the trustees have a fiduciary responsibility for investment of the plan's assets. One advantage of self-directed plans is that they offer more flexibility for the individual participants, who may have different investment needs, philosophies, or horizons. A second advantage is that, if this arrangement meets certain DOL criteria defined in ERISA Section 404(c), the trustees have some protection from fiduciary responsibility for the participants' investment decisions.[34]

A major disadvantage to self-directed plans is that they are usually more expensive and more cumbersome to administer. Second, some of the participants may not be knowledgeable regarding investments and require some basic investment education. The practice should exercise caution in providing this information, because doing so can subject the practice, the trustees, and other fiduciaries to legal risk – that is, providing investment *information* could be construed to be investment *advice*. ERISA does provide some safe harbors regarding the provision of investment information, such as use of advice created with a computer model and advice given under an arrangement in which the provider's fees cannot vary based on the investment option selected. The safe harbor includes many additional requirements, such as giving notice and an annual audit by an independent auditor.[35] Because of the risks involved in providing this information, a practice should use due diligence in providing investment information to its participants. This includes having a formal contract with a provider who is knowledgeable in both investments and ERISA requirements.[36] It is often inadvisable for an employer to provide advice to employees regarding their retirement plan investments.

Selective Plan Considerations

Loans to Participants

Some plans allow loans to participants. These loans must carry a reasonable rate of interest, be sufficiently secured, and be granted on a nondiscriminatory basis. The participants must repay the loans under a reasonable repayment schedule, including payments made at least quarterly, with level amortization. (Handling repayment through authorized payroll deduction often works well.) The repayment period of a loan cannot exceed five years, except when the loan relates to the acquisition of the participant's personal residence.

Finally, a participant cannot borrow more than the lesser of $50,000 or 50 percent of the participant's vested balance; otherwise, the proceeds will be treated as a distribution.[37]

The obvious advantage to allowing participant loans is that it provides a mechanism for participants to access their retirement funds to meet an emergency or other financial need. In some instances, employees who cannot borrow from a plan may terminate their employment in order to receive a distribution.

Two disadvantages are that (1) administering participant loans adds time and complexity to managing the plan, and (2) by taking loans against their balance, employees potentially reduce the amount of funds available for their retirement.

Top-Heavy Considerations

When a plan fails DOL- and IRS-mandated nondiscrimination testing, it may be classified as "top heavy." A defined contribution plan is generally considered top heavy if, as of the determination date, 60 percent or more of the aggregate account balances accrue to key employees. For a SEP plan, this determination may be based on either aggregate account balances or aggregate contributions.[38]

Medical practice plans are likely to be considered top heavy. If so, regulations require certain minimum benefits and vesting requirements in the plan. If the plan is not top heavy, then normal vesting and funding requirements apply. Most 401(k) plans in smaller medical practices are almost always established using the safe harbor provisions described previously to eliminate any potential refunding of physician-owner deferrals.

Eligibility and Vesting

A qualified plan may have certain age and service limitations as a condition for participation in the plan, except that plans cannot generally exclude employees over the age of 21 who have completed at least one year of service. Special rules may apply for employees that work less than a full-time schedule and those with breaks in service.

Once an employee becomes eligible, he or she must begin participating no later than the earlier of the next plan entry date or six months after the date s/he meets eligibility requirements. To satisfy this condition, plans often have two plan entry dates per year – one on the first day of the plan year and one six months later.

Once an employee begins participating, the plan's vesting provisions will determine what percentage of an employee's balance is nonforfeitable (for example, if the employee terminates employment). An employee's own contributions, such as 401(k) deferrals, are never subject to vesting. In addition, any funding to the plan under the safe harbor provisions is not subject to vesting. The law generally allows for vesting of other employer contributions over a three- to seven-year period, with certain minimum amounts vested at the end of each year.

One notable exception to the eligibility and vesting rules is that a plan may require an employee to have two years of service to be eligible to participate in the plan; in this situation, however, the plan must provide 100-percent vesting immediately. The two-years-of-service option is only available for the employer contributions; the plan must still allow for employee contributions after one year. This two-year eligibility and immediate vesting option may be beneficial for practices that have high turnover rates for recently hired employees.[39]

Contribution Formula

Defined contribution plans need to specify how contributions are determined and allocated. This formula must follow certain rules regarding maximum contribution amounts and generally not discriminate in favor of employees with high salaries. For money purchase pension plans, this formula is especially crucial because it results in a mandatory contribution to the plan each year. If the practice sets this percentage too high, it could create cash flow problems or result in lower physician salaries. If the practice sets this percentage too low, the physicians and employees would have less accumulation in their retirement funds.

Defined contribution plans are generally designed to maximize the contribution of the physicians-owners and balance that with the desired funding level for the staff. This design typically includes a 401(k) deferral option, an employer match, a nonelective contribution that satisfies the safe harbor provisions, and a discretionary profit-sharing contribution (designed to maximize physician-owner contributions). Notice requirements (discussed later in this chapter) allow the practice to satisfy the nondiscrimination testing.[40]

Although qualified plans may not generally discriminate in favor of highly compensated employees, both defined benefit and defined contribution plans may coordinate the plan contribution/ benefit formula with payments the practice makes into the Social Security retirement system. This has the effect of reducing the contribution or benefit for the compensation an employee receives that is below the Social Security taxable wage base.[41] These plans are typically referred to as integrated plans, which means integrated with the Social Security wage base. Another popular design is referred to as a cross-tested plan, which is based, in part, on the ages of the plan participants. The complexities of this plan design are beyond the scope of this text but are worthy of consideration as part of a practice's plan design.

Because actuaries determine the contribution for traditional defined benefit plans, practices do not generally need to devise a formula for these contributions. The practice does, however, need to determine the level of benefit it wishes to provide.

Plan Administration and Maintenance

After the plan is in place, the practice must fulfill its responsibilities under the plan, such as ensuring that various reports are filed and distributed on a regular basis. This normally involves hiring a third-party administrator, but the practice and the trustees are ultimately responsible for ensuring that these functions are in compliance with all applicable laws. The practice administrator generally coordinates internal compliance and related communications with third-party vendors. Employees must complete enrollment forms in connection with their plan participation, which typically include their election to participate, their investment direction (if self-directed), and a designation of beneficiary form. Contributions, including employee deferrals, must be deposited into the plan on a regular basis. Finally, the practice should continually evaluate its plan design and investment process and performance to ensure that the plan continues to satisfy the goals of the physician-owners and the employees.

Legal Documents

Continual updates and modifications of tax laws and other legislation require that plan documents be reviewed at least annually. In the case of a prototype plan, the company that sponsors the prototype generally will coordinate all necessary amendments and communications with participants and governmental agencies. If the practice has an individually designed plan, it will need its attorney or other retirement plan professional to draft the necessary amendments to the plan and complete the other necessary actions. If the practice has an ongoing relationship with this attorney or outside advisor, he or she will generally inform the practice when these amendments are required.

Practices with a safe harbor 401(k) plan should provide notice to the participants of the intention to fund the plan and the method of contribution to be used (as previously discussed). This is generally necessary for the plan to meet the safe harbor requirements and eliminate the nondiscrimination testing.

Reporting Requirements

Participants are legally required to receive adequate plan information on a regular basis. Initially, they should be provided with a summary plan description (an abbreviated version of the legal documents that describe how the plan operates on a day-to-day basis). They should also receive appropriate notification when the plan is amended or restated. If the practice has a safe harbor 401(k) plan, it will also need to provide the participants notice each year as described above.

Plan participants should receive regular statements that summarize the financial transactions occurring in their accounts, including employer and employee funding, as well as transfers between investments and income (realized and unrealized gains and losses). They must also receive a copy of the plan's annual report, which is typically prepared by the third-party administrator.[42]

For most plans, the practice will have to file IRS Form 5500, "Annual Return/Report of Employee Benefit Plan." Although this is an IRS form, it is a consolidated return that meets the requirements of the IRS, the DOL, and the PBGC.[43]

Administrative Services, Record-Keeping, and Investment Management

In most cases, an employer/plan sponsor retains the services of a third-party administrator to assist in complying with the legal requirements of the plan. Typically, the third-party administrator completes the compliance services required for the plan, including any testing or reporting requirements. The practice should take particular care in selecting a firm to perform those services to ensure compliance with regulatory agencies and also to receive proper service and expertise. Depending on where and how the assets are invested, the third-party administrator may or may not serve as the record-keeper and provide the necessary quarterly or annual participant statements.

Larger group practices may hire accountants and actuaries to provide these functions internally. Practices should compare the costs of using third parties with those of hiring qualified employees. Even practices that handle plan administration services internally may have to hire external third-party administrators or actuaries to provide consulting services for the group in order to ensure compliance.

New Participant Paperwork

Within the 30- to 90-day period prior to the time employees become participants in the plan, they should receive certain information regarding the plan. The new participants will need a copy of the summary plan description and, if applicable, any safe harbor notices.

Each participant must complete a form designating his or her beneficiary, which is provided by the service provider who drafts the plan document. In general, married individuals must name their spouse as their beneficiary unless the spouse signs a form that provides consent otherwise. This can avoid potential problems if the participant dies. For example, a participant might name a child as a beneficiary without considering who the guardian might be or list a group such as "all my children" rather than providing specific names.

As discussed earlier, if the practice has a 401(k) plan, the participant has to complete a form selecting the amount of his or her deferral contribution and authorizing the related payroll deduction. For self-directed plans, the practice may need documentation of the participants' selected investments.

Contributions

The practice has to ensure that it deposits all plan contributions in a timely manner. This includes employer contributions and employee contributions, such as deferrals and loan repayments.

The practice must generally pay employer contributions to the plan no later than the due date of its tax return, including extensions. For corporate entities, the due date is two and one-half months following the end of the year. For partnerships, limited liability entities, and sole proprietorships, this due date is three and one-half months following the end of the year. All entities may apply for an automatic six-month extension. (For a discussion regarding cash flow issues regarding timing of retirement plan contributions, see the *Body of Knowledge Review: Financial Management* book.)

ERISA regulations require that the practice deposit employee contributions as soon as possible, but no later than the 15th business day of the month following the month in which these amounts were withheld from the employees' pay. In at least one court case, the court was not lenient: an employer that failed to deposit elective deposits within two business days after they were withheld was deemed to have made a fiduciary breech. To confirm that employee deferrals are deposited timely, Form 5500 contains a question on whether these payments have been made in a timely manner.

The DOL is more strict about deposits of employee loan repayments to the plan. They have stated that the deferral deposit standard of the 15th business day of the following month rule does not hold; these should be deposited in the plan as soon as they can be reasonably segregated from the practice's assets.[44]

Distributions

The practice must properly handle participant distributions. Most of the time these are distributions to terminated participants or their beneficiaries; however, the practice may also have to make distributions to current employees who have reached the age at which they must take required distributions (currently 70½).

A practice should pay distributions to terminated employees in accordance with its plan documents and the applicable regulations. It should provide a notice to the terminated employee or beneficiary explaining the tax rules regarding the distribution, such as the roll-over option and federal income tax withholding on taxable distributions. The IRS has written a model notice that employers may use for this purpose. Third-party administrators or other advisors usually provide the required forms and notices.

The participant or beneficiary may elect a direct rollover of the contribution to an IRA or other qualified retirement plan, and avoid paying current income taxes on the distribution.

If the participant or beneficiary elects to receive the distribution, the practice must generally withhold 20 percent of the distribution as federal income taxes. Unless the participant or beneficiary rolls the gross amount of this distribution over to an IRA or other qualified plan within 60 days, the distribution will be taxable income to that individual. Participants who are younger than 59½ years of age and are not disabled must generally pay an additional 10 percent early distribution penalty.

No distributions should be made from the plan without signed distribution documents from the participant. In most cases, the third-party administrator or record-keeper assists the employer in the distribution process.

■ Plan Monitoring and Ongoing Assessment

Plan trustees should ensure that the appropriate tools are in place to monitor the continued successful operation of the retirement plan. A practice should regularly evaluate plan investment performance, such as by comparing the return on investment to major indices.

The trustees' fiduciary responsibility includes proper and prudent investment of plan assets, even when it uses outside investment managers. The key to monitoring and assessment of the plan is the process used, not necessarily the end result.

Tax laws can change, as can the practice's needs. The trustees should periodically evaluate the structure of their existing plan to determine whether it best meets their current needs.

Chapter 5 **Training for Medical Providers, Employees, and Students**

EVERY MEDICAL PRACTICE, if it wants to gain market share and become or remain successful, must provide its employees with continuing education. Whether it is pursued through internal means (staff meetings, training sessions, etc.) or through external means (association meetings, consultants, paid training sessions), continuing education builds a solid foundation of knowledge to better perform jobs. Every practice needs its employees to have continuing-education updates on safety (Occupational Safety and Health Administration, universal precautions, fire prevention, and the like) and compliance (e.g., the Health Insurance Portability and Accountability Act, correct billing practices, and so forth), along with updates on technology and regulatory changes (e.g., Medicare, Medicaid, state laws). Continuing education may also be needed to keep an employee licensed or registered in a particular profession.

The medical practice needs to determine, in advance, what it will pay for training for the employee. Employee training can be very costly, but is usually worth the investment. The costs can usually be higher if the practice *doesn't* invest in its employees – through lost productivity, citations, violation fees, fines, and other risk management issues.

For training to be effective, it must address a positive environment for learning, the quality of the materials provided, employee motivation and incentives to be trained, and adult learning models based on the group being trained. Training must be staffed by trained professionals as opposed to experts in content material and by people who can teach adults and provide different learning modes. Training is an investment in the medical practice, and its results can be tied to the medical practice's performance.

◼ Organizational Operations/Practices

Philosophy of Training and Development

Medical practices need to be aware of the ongoing changes facing the practice of medicine. To keep up with the changes in reimbursement, coding, managed care, compliance, and clinical practice, the employer must provide the employee with appropriate formats for learning. With the proliferation of technological advances, the medical practice executive should look at new options to improve results and outcomes. The medical practice and its employees are becoming more sophisticated consumers and are demanding better access to information. The employee demands more professional development opportunities, better access to those resources, and greater flexibility to learn.

The human capital for the medical practice is very important, and this recognition is critical in developing resources to meet the needs of the current work force. The medical practice must be proactive in recruiting, managing, and retaining the best people to meet the organization's mission, goals, and objectives. To this end, it is critical for the medical practice to ensure that its employees have the necessary skills, resources, and abilities to perform their jobs. The diversity and variety of training opportunities will help the employee to see how the medical practice culture is conveyed through its training resources.

Training Value to Organization

The value of training to the organization can be measured through integration with appropriate evaluation tools. Evaluation tools are quick and objective ways to identify the strengths and weaknesses of the learning done. Evaluation is drawn from the employee evaluation, participant learning, achievement of the behavior change sought, and the overall impact on the organization. Accomplishment of these areas provides the demonstrated value of training and shows how it can impact the medical practice's revenue and profit, employee satisfaction, market share, and patient satisfaction.

Present Cost vs. Future Investment

Training is a budgeted line item, and its impact is measurable by future outcomes. For example, a medical assistant who performs charge entry must be familiar with Current Procedural Terminology (CPT®) and ICD-9 codes and needs to have knowledge of appropriate documentation for billing. Effective training will help the employee to question mistakes and capture possible lost charges or incorrectly coded charge tickets. A medical biller may be able to handle billing error follow-up better if he or she is trained on the correct coding edits and how to communicate with front-end staff on how to avoid these kinds of errors. This training will lead to faster payment and fewer errors to track. The cost to handle errors will be less, so the staff can focus more energy on doing things correctly than on fixing mistakes. Failure to provide training up front will result in poorer performance and outcomes in the future.

The medical practice executive should plan for employee training and determine who is eligible, how training needs are determined, and how those services are obtained. Reimbursement may be prepaid or paid after successful completion of the program. Tuition coverage may be a separate benefit to provide employee training or may be used to allow an employee to pursue higher education in a field that would benefit the medical group, such as business, nursing, or allied health.

Scheduling for Training

Freeing up staff to be trained is a logistics challenge. Time must be budgeted to allow staff to be appropriately oriented and trained. Creative scheduling and flexible staffing are needed to accommodate and allow all staff to be trained.

Replacement Schedules

Depending on the size of the medical group, staff may be specifically hired to cover schedules of other staff when they are being trained. Replacement schedules allow staff members to be focused on the training at hand with the knowledge and comfort that their shifts are being appropriately covered.

Release Time

A medical group needs to determine under what circumstances an employee will be allowed company time or paid release time to attend an educational program.

Overtime Considerations

Although the goal is to use part-time and as-needed staff to cover staff being trained, there are times when staff will need to work overtime to accommodate the training needs of the organization. Overtime may need to be used for large-scale training projects, such as computer conversions, implementation of an electronic health record (EHR), or new equipment.

Paid Attendance, Meeting Time, and Continuing Medical Education Policy

Paid attendance may be specifically defined and there may be a cap on dollars or days available for training. For example, a physician may be given one week of continuing medical education days paid by the medical group not to exceed $3,000 per calendar year. This guideline helps every employee to manage expenses and time away from the practice appropriately.

◼ Types of Training

Training content determination is a multidisciplinary group process. Usually groups identify more topics and issues than what can possibly be covered. Teams can help prioritize topics and level of detail needed for training, and this, in turn, largely determines the type of training to be pursued.

Orientation

All employees receive a general orientation to the organization. Usually, there is a general overview of the medical group, its practices and policies, and then a departmental orientation. These orientations can take hours or weeks to complete, depending on the complexity and level of detail needed for the employee.

Supervisory/Management

A management development program that creates a guide and/or template for the new manager to follow allows the manager to be aware of those areas that he or she needs to know within the organization prior to completing a full orientation.

Technical/Skills

Depending on the nature of the job, an employer may train the staff on technical and skill-based employment functions. Or they may expect a core level of technical and skill-based knowledge, but train the employee specifically on the organizational-based skill needed for the job.

Career Development

An employer may support an employee through career development opportunities. The employee may be afforded the opportunity to seek additional training and career advancement at the employer's expense. The long-term expectations of the employee must be clearly stated prior to the employee seeking these educational opportunities.

Certification

Certification allows the employee to demonstrate a core competency or knowledge in a specific field of study. Certification provides acknowledgment of skill, knowledge, education, and proficiency achieved in an area. Sometimes certification is required for initial employment or to continue being employed in the medical group.

Cross-Training

Cross-training a staff member allows the staff to be flexible in staffing schedules and allows staff to take time off without the worry of how the employee's tasks will be performed during the employee's absence. It also allows multiple people to be involved in a task and provide creative suggestions and ideas on how to improve a system or process. However, if cross-training is not done well, a person may assume a task and perform the task poorly through learned bad habits or behaviors. Cross-training must be continuously evaluated to ensure that employees provide quality in the work performed.

■ Adult Learning Styles

Employee training programs can be developed and implemented by the medical practice or can be outsourced to other agencies, schools, or organizations that focus on specific topics or issues. Training programs can take on many different forms to help the adult learner. An adult learner generally approaches learning differently from a young student. The adult usually is more self-guided in learning, brings more experience to the learning process, expects more from the learning experience, and will challenge any learning that doesn't make sense.

Learning by Doing

Many people learn best by doing. A medical assistant can learn all about how and why and under what circumstances to draw blood and about the tools needed to perform the function, but there is nothing like practicing on oneself and others to learn. Learning by doing can be invaluable as long as there is a written plan to demonstrate proficiency and competency in a learned function.

Didactic Teaching

Common classroom settings, which nearly every American has experienced at some time through formal education, provide a lesson plan, reading, class interaction, possible homework, and a test to measure whether the adult learner has mastered the skill or body of knowledge.

Mentoring and Coaching

Mentoring is a method of supporting a new employee to learn new tasks and duties from an exceptionally performing employee. Sometimes mentoring supports a current employee who is interested in learning new job tasks or functions. Mentoring must be carefully planned because some employees are exceptional employees but poor mentors or trainers. Some people know how to perform a job well but do not know how to show someone else how to do the same job. A mentor should be an active listener who is patient, willing to explain things repetitively, and able to break down job tasks into smaller segments and describe how they fit together. Many times, a mentor can become the company trainer or coach.

Coaching provides individual one-on-one attention to an employee needing greater supervision and encouragement. Coaching is a cyclical process that works with the adult learner and determines what kind of support the employee needs depending on the personal traits of the employee. The coaching support will depend on what part of the cycle the employee is in with respect to the task being mastered and learned. Usually, the new employee is a beginner and is usually enthusiastic to learn a new skill, but may be apprehensive about making mistakes. The learner needs clear instructions, constant feedback, emotional support, and praise when a task is learned well.

The next level of coaching is providing a lot of technical and emotional support for the employee so he or she is not discouraged from performing a task because of mistakes made. Also, poor technique should not become learned; bad habits can be difficult to break. Once the employee has learned the new skill, the coach provides guidance to reinforce the skill learned until the employee has mastered the skill and has become an expert. At that point, the employee needs little direction or support. The employee embraces the new task, takes ownership of the task, and begins to take on new tasks and responsibilities, and the coach can begin to work with the employee on new skills. Coaching helps to build employee confidence and affirms that the employee is performing aspects of the job correctly. Coaching also provides positive reinforcement of a job well done.

Self-Directed Learning

With the proliferation of computer technology, numerous self-directed learning modules can support an employee to learn new tasks and functions independently. These programs comprise reading, example problems, case studies, and questions to answer prior to taking a test. A self-directed program can be very effective for a well-motivated, organized adult. If the adult struggles with self-motivation, organizing and/or prioritizing workload, and/or using computers or reading booklets, a self-directed program may not work well.

Group Interaction

Providing a forum for group interaction can be a powerful and effective way for an employee to learn. Group interaction can promote personal growth, teach professional skills, and provide a cost-effective method to learn tasks and skills. The learning can be customized based on the particular group brought together. The group interaction can be based on small work groups, large forums, workshops, or even computer online Internet classes with dialogue forums.

Training Formats

Computer Media

Computer-based training allows the employee to use specific software on a self-directed basis to learn a new skill. The employee must have a basic level of comfort with computers to perform these tasks. Videos were very popular for training purposes during the last two decades; now, interactive videos in a VHS or DVD format are available on Internet and intranet sites. The low cost for this technology, when compared to staff travel and per diem costs, has made it a convenient venue for training.

Interactive Training

Interactive training allows the employee to participate in the process and learn by doing. A phlebotomy training class that allows the employee to practice drawing blood is more effective than just reading a book. Interactive training may involve a "skills lab" where employees can work in a simulated setting (e.g., patient exam room, telephone for customer service skills).

Role Playing

Role-playing exercises allow the employee to test practical knowledge learned in a real-life situation, but in a manner that is safe and protected. For example, a manager may learn how to have a "critical conversation" with an employee about poor work performance. The role play would allow the manager to talk with a trainer who pretends to be the disgruntled employee. Trying out different situations allows the manager to see whether the learned skills can be applied practically in a situation. The trainer provides feedback and constructive input on areas that can be improved in this situation.

Lecturer

A lecture or speaker presentation is another common educational format that is popular with large groups of people. The speaker may use overheads or handouts to cover the material and allow questions either during the presentation or at the end.

Group Discussion

A group discussion allows people to ask questions and hear different perspectives about an issue or topic. The group discussion may be focused on a series of questions that are asked of the group after the presentation of materials. Getting the group involved helps to affirm the topic and reinforce the knowledge.

Books

Books, workbooks, resource manuals, training manuals, and other printed material have been the most traditional resources for training. However, with the development of the Internet and Web-based applications, more books are being placed online.

Education Technology Online

Educational resources are now available online. A participant can log on to any computer with Internet access and take a class. The technology will monitor modules completed, tests taken, and completion of the training program. These applications make training much more accessible, convenient, and flexible. Many applications provide the participant with videos to watch and even provide opportunities to submit information and written materials for the reviewer to evaluate.

Outsourced Training

The use of outsourcing vs. an in-house training staff depends on the needs of the organization. Usually, the larger the organization, the more likely the medical group will pursue an in-house training staff. Smaller medical groups do not have the ability to hire someone full time to handle in-house needs.

An outsourced training program can be efficient, cost-effective, and provide a strong service level for the customer because the client provides these services routinely to a large group of employees. Outsourcing allows the medical practice to focus its energy on other aspects of the operations. Every physician practice has a limited number of human resources staff, whose services are focused on serving the employees and improving service excellence. With outsourced training, a physician group can use the best practices, systems, and educational venues with a smaller investment than creating, maintaining, and improving an in-house training program.

For certain areas, however, as a medical group expands and grows, there is value in having an in-house staff. A medical practice executive may bring certain training functions in-house (e.g., computer training, compliance, and safety training), but continue to outsource other training functions (e.g., cardiopulmonary resuscitation, CPT training). Regardless of the decision made, a physician practice must evaluate and discern how in-house and outsourced training will be used to educate employees.

Training the Trainer

Training the trainer allows a medical group to have one person or a group of people trained on a specific application or area of training and then bring that information back to the organization for on-site training and implementation. It can be project specific (e.g., EHR implementation), department specific (e.g., nursing orientation), or organization specific (e.g., information technology, technology, computer, and clinical training). The trainer needs to be comfortable with using adult learning principles and focus on a program that develops objectives, selects the appropriate training method, develops training aids, and uses facilitation and problem-solving skills. In addition, a mechanism should be in place to evaluate the training sessions.

◼ Conclusion

Whatever the venue or approach toward training, medical groups should develop a process that will achieve its desired outcomes. The employee must be made aware of the topic, acquire the knowledge, change behavior, and achieve desired results. The medical group should improve the quality of learning for its employees and reduce course work and training time in an environment of limited resources. Even though more resources are available now than ever before, with the proliferation of computer training, the numerous options are confusing and it is difficult to stay focused on those core competencies that need to be achieved.

Training will continue to be a challenge for all medical practice executives until there is a focus on improving performance to achieve practice goals as opposed to solely increasing skill and knowledge. It is common for medical groups to assume that training is the outcome or solution without fully understanding the cause of the problems being addressed.

Chapter 6 **Complying with Employment Laws and Regulatory Standards**

HUMAN RESOURCE POLICIES provide a framework for both the medical practice and the employee. These policies allow the medical practice to direct its employee relations and articulate what is expected, and the policies should prevent any misunderstandings about employer policies.

Employees often do not know their rights and responsibilities and may receive bad advice from co-workers or friends. An employee handbook that spells out the medical practice's procedures and policies can help provide each employee with guidance on what is considered an "acceptable" practice and well within the law.

Smaller medical practices may not have the range of written policies and procedures that a larger practice will. Regardless of practice size, the medical practice executive is responsible for ensuring that all appropriate laws and regulations are observed and followed. Failure to do so may result in inconsistent and noncompliant practices and cause for a potential lawsuit.

Employment law is complex and requires a keen awareness to ensure compliance. A medical practice executive may need support from an attorney or human resources

(HR) consultant to ensure compliance with all appropriate laws. A periodic external review of current practices to ensure compliance with the law will demonstrate a commitment toward compliance. Written policies should be reviewed by legal counsel to ensure that they reflect applicable federal, state, and local requirements.

A well-run medical practice will be up to date on the various labor relations issues that may impact a practice. Whether this is done through an experienced human resources professional, outside legal counsel, or the medical practice executive's own efforts, he or she should be knowledgeable on a range of issues, from requirements on minimum wage, workers' compensation, unemployment compensation, to unions, collective bargaining, and fair employment practices.

■ Employee Handbook

Every medical practice should have an employee handbook, which is given to each employee with the expectation that he or she signs a statement indicating its receipt and agreement to abide by its policies. The following topics would typically be included in an employee handbook:

- *Medical practice welcome*. Welcome statement from a key leader; a disclaimer that the information in the handbook is not all-inclusive;

- *Introduction*. Mission statement, career opportunities, and code of conduct;

- *Employment*. Equal employment opportunity; employment eligibility; eligibility for employment; nepotism; criminal convictions; violence and use of weapons; alcohol, drugs and illegal substance abuse; sexual and other types of harassment; employee evaluations; access to one's personnel file;

- *Policies and procedures*. Attendance; parking; work schedule requirements; bulletin boards; time cards; lunch and other breaks; dress code; compensation and overtime; taxes, FICA (Federal Insurance Contributions Act), and Medicare taxes;

performance and evaluation reviews; reporting personal information changes; gifts, entertainment, and meals; visitors; personal property; personal safety; smoking; drug testing; noncompete and nondisclosure agreement;

- *Company property*. Confidential information security; office supplies; postage and company accounts; phone systems; voice mail and personal calls; conservation and recycling;

- *Computer-related policies*. Computers and related equipment; use of the Internet and intranet; use of e-mail and electronic communications;

- *Policies for leave of absence*. Eligibility, personal and sick leave; unpaid leave; absence under the Family and Medical Leave Act of 1993 (FMLA); jury and military duty;

- *Benefits*. Health and dental insurance; pension; life insurance; and

- *Discipline policies*. Progressive discipline; violation of company policy; termination of employment.

The Medical Group Management Association (MGMA) offers a customizable *Staff Handbook for Medical Practices* with an accompanying CD.

General Regulations

Wages and Benefits

From a legal perspective the medical practice follows the federal Fair Labor Standards Act, which requires a minimum wage of $6.55 per hour. This act also requires equal pay for equal work regardless of gender. Some states have enacted higher minimum wage requirements, but most medical practices pay employees more than the minimum wage.

A medical practice may not restrict benefits for employees of a like group. Benefits must be administered fairly and consistently. For example, if health insurance is available for full-time nonexempt

staff, a medical practice may not indicate that one medical recep-
tionist may have health insurance and another one cannot because
that employee has insurance with a spouse. The benefit must be
offered to all eligible employees. It is up to the employee to determine whether he or she wants, or is even eligible for, that benefit.

Performance

Performance or lack of performance and how that evaluation is
communicated with the employee could result in an unsatisfied
employee. If the employee can demonstrate that the performance
review is discriminatory or has violated a certain law, the medical
practice must be confident that its practices and process comply
with the law.

Many lawsuits surround employees contesting a disciplinary
action process that results in termination. It is critical that the medical practice have a written process that is consistent with the law
and is administered fairly and consistently.

Safety and Health

Every medical practice must keep its employees safe from harm. The
physician credo to "do no harm" to the patient must be extended
to the employee in the workplace. The medical practice executive
should work diligently toward employee and patient safety. The
practice environment must be safe and comply with Occupational
Safety and Health Administration (OSHA) laws as well as with local
zoning or building codes.

Fraud and Abuse

The U.S. Office of Inspector General carries out a broad range of
duties nationally through audits, investigations, and inspections to
protect the U.S. Department of Health and Human Services programs
and the beneficiaries of those programs. It has developed guidelines
for individual and small medical practices toward the development and implementation of a voluntary compliance program that
promotes adherence to any and all federal health care program
requirements. Every medical practice has a duty and responsibility
to ensure that its physicians and employees are knowledgeable and

committed to following the rules and regulations of the federal government and that they know what those rules are. The guidelines include the following:

- Designating a compliance officer;
- Implementing compliance through written and well-communicated standards;
- Having practice-specific education and training;
- Communicating appropriately with employees, physicians, and others;
- Performing internal monitoring and auditing;
- Responding to compliance issues with appropriate correction action; and
- Enforcing sanctions for noncompliance.

Nondiscrimination

Medical practices may have a nondiscrimination statement that would prohibit discrimination in all of its activities on the basis of certain classes such as race, color, national origin, sex, religion, age, disability, sexual orientation, and marital or family status. Persons with disabilities who require other means for medical practice communication information, such as interpretation services, should contact the medical practice executive. Also, the medical practice executive should offer the person the ability to file a complaint of discrimination by providing an address and/or telephone number for the person to contact, if warranted. The medical practice usually would provide a statement in its internal publications that states "ABC Medical Practice is an equal opportunity provider and employer."

Payroll Records

Every medical group needs to keep records on its payroll practices. Based on the common saying, "If it's not documented, it wasn't done," medical practices need to have employees document the hours worked in the practice. Payroll procedures and policies should be established to ensure that a fair, consistent, and legal process is followed in paying employees the correct amount for the exact hours worked. There are particular laws that govern payroll practices, including that nonsalaried employees are to be compensated for overtime, and that time cards are properly completed and signed off by employees. In many organizations, inaccurately completed time cards can result in termination.

Employment at Will

Many U.S. states have an "employment at will" policy, which means that an employer may hire or fire an employee at will without any resource or reason. However, because of the numerous employment laws and regulations, an employer may have to prove that terminating an employee was not due to discrimination. As a result, the employer may need to indicate specifically why the employee was terminated.

State and Local Laws on Sexual Orientation

Sexual orientation laws have been developed by some states and localities, but not federally. A medical practice should be fully aware of its state laws and the respective requirements placed on the employer. In New York, for example, the Sexual Orientation Non-Discrimination Act of 2002 prohibits discrimination on the basis of actual or perceived sexual orientation in employment, housing, public accommodations, education, credit, and the exercise of civil rights. This latter protected category was newly added to various state laws, including New York's Human Rights Law, Civil Rights Law, and Education Law. Although a medical practice may choose to follow a certain law even if it isn't required in its particular location, it must follow those laws and their administration in those states where it does apply. This involves the medical practice executive knowing not just that the state law exists, but also how it is interpreted and implemented in that state. Usually, when a law is passed, numerous legal firms and HR consultants are available to provide advice on how to follow the new law.

Licensure/Certification

Certain medical professions require licensure or certification. The medical practice executive should ensure that the affected employees are appropriately licensed or certified and that their licenses are updated accordingly. For example, a physician's medical license is state specific and requires renewal on a periodic basis. The medical practice executive needs to keep the physician's updated medical license on file because that is a requirement for employment. Failure to do so could result in a medical provider administering care without a license, and the concomitant sanctions against the practice for allowing the provider to do so.

Record-Keeping

Keeping accurate and timely employee records and files is necessary to maintain a well-run practice. From updated addresses and emergency contacts to completed tax forms and signed disciplinary action paperwork, the medical practice executive should provide diligent maintenance of employee records. Practical issues follow if the records are not kept up to date. In an emergency situation in which the medical practice building is without electrical power and the practice will be closed, employees need to be informed of the closure. If telephone numbers are not updated, a problem exists for contacting employees in a timely manner. Personnel records must also be up to date in case of a medical problem with an employee, such as fainting while on the job; without current records, it may take life-saving time to determine the possible reason for the fainting, such as an insulin attack.

▪ Specific Legislation

Americans with Disabilities Act of 1990

The ADA prohibits discrimination and guarantees equal opportunity for persons with disabilities in employment. A medical practice must make reasonable accommodation for a disabled employee to perform his or her job. In addition, the ADA specifies services for nonemployees, including having handicapped-accessible restrooms and providing access to interpretation services for deaf patients or patients requiring a language interpreter.

The Family and Medical Leave Act of 1993

The FMLA requires covered employers to provide up to 12 weeks of unpaid, job-protected leave to "eligible" employees for certain family and medical reasons. Medical practice employees are eligible if they have worked for the medical practice for more than one year, for 1,250 hours over the previous 12 months, and if there are at least 50 employees within the medical group within 75 miles of the practice's main office (some employees may work off-site or at satellite clinics, but these must be within a 75-mile radius). In addition, FMLA allows employees to take leave on an intermittent basis or to work a reduced schedule under certain circumstances. This far-reaching legislation has tremendous employment impact for larger medical groups with more than 50 employees but does not impact smaller medical groups. By being legally required to hold a person's job for up to 12 weeks, the larger medical practice is challenged to find adequate and appropriate coverage during this time frame.

Occupational Safety and Health Act of 1970

The Occupational Safety and Health Act protects employees from harm on the job and has established a nationwide, federal program to protect the workforce from job-related death, injury, and illness. OSHA was developed within the Department of Labor to administer the act. OSHA has significant impact on a medical practice, especially in the areas of responsibility that include policies on blood-borne pathogens, emergency response, hearing safety, lockout/tagout, respiratory safety, lead safety, fire safety, office ergonomics, personal protective equipment, material safety data sheets, and right to know for hazard communication materials. A medical practice must be fully aware and compliant with OSHA regulations at the workplace. Complying with OSHA will help to provide the workplace and employees with a safe environment in which to work. A medical practice must have knowledgeable people well versed on OSHA, its requirements, and practical implementation of those requirements.

Civil Rights Act of 1964/Title VII

The Civil Rights Act was passed to provide guidance on discriminatory practices, including discrimination due to race, color, religion, gender, or national origin. Title VII of the act covers specific information about such discrimination and other unlawful employment practices.

Immigration Reform and Control Act of 1986

The Immigration Reform and Control Act controls unauthorized U.S. immigration by instituting employer sanctions and penalties if aliens are hired who are not authorized to work in the United States. Every new hire in a medical practice needs to complete an I-9 form documenting through two approved source documents that he or she is not an illegal alien. A medical practice executive cannot cut corners by failing to have new employees complete this form.

National Labor Relations Act of 1935

The NLRA guarantees workers the right to join unions without fear of management retaliation. The National Labor Relations Board enforces this right and bans employers from committing unfair labor practices that would deter organizing or prevent workers from negotiating a union contract. Employees have the right to self-organization, to be part of labor organizations, and to collective bargaining and its activities.

Equal Pay Act of 1963

The Equal Pay Act is part of the Fair Labor Standards Act of 1938, enforced by the Equal Employment Opportunity Commission. It prohibits sex-based wage discrimination between men and women in the same medical practice who perform duties under similar working conditions. If a court finds that the practice is in violation of this act, the judge can fine the group up to $10,000 and/or send the responsible party (e.g., the owner or the medical practice executive) to jail for up to six months. Gender should not be taken into consideration when paying an employee for work done in the medical practice.

Age Discrimination in Employment Act of 1967

The Age Discrimination in Employment Act prohibits employment discrimination against persons 40 years of age or older. This act is meant to promote employment of older people based on ability rather than age, to prevent arbitrary age discrimination in employment, and to help medical practices find ways to address employment problems stemming from age issues. When hiring an employee, age should not be taken into consideration for older workers unless it can be demonstrated that age is a factor in preventing the employee from adequately performing the job.

Vocational Rehabilitation Act

In 1920, the U.S. Congress passed the Smith-Fess Act promoting states to give rehabilitation services to disabled veterans. Succeeding legislation has expanded the services and those who can receive them. The Vocational Rehabilitation program now operates under the authority of the Rehabilitation Act of 1973. Medical practice executives can work with agencies to determine how they can help support this program including ways to provide potential candidates with jobs.

Vietnam-Era Veterans' Readjustment Assistance Act of 1974

The Vietnam-Era Veterans' Readjustment Assistance Act requires that employers with federal contracts or subcontracts of $25,000 or more provide equal opportunity for Vietnam-era veterans, special disabled veterans, and certain veterans who served on active duty. Although this law may not apply to medical practices, the medical group must be aware of the circumstances under which it may apply.

Pregnancy Discrimination Act of 1978

The U.S. Pregnancy Discrimination Act indicates that discrimination on the basis of pregnancy, childbirth, or related medical conditions is unlawful under Title VII of the Civil Rights Act. A pregnant woman should be evaluated regarding her ability or inability to work and should not be terminated, be refused employment, or, conversely, be promoted because of a pregnancy.

Affirmative Action

Affirmative action is the set of public policies designed to help eliminate discrimination based on race, color, religion, sex, or national origin. The medical practice executive can request that all potential employees complete a form indicating their backgrounds, which are independently summarized to demonstrate that the practice is considering all potential candidates regardless of race, color, religion, sex, or national origin. Sometimes a practice will list that it is an "affirmative action employer" to demonstrate its commitment to diversity.

◼ Supervisory Training on Legal Requirements

A medical practice cannot assume that every new supervisor is knowledgeable about the various laws and requirements of the medical practice. An orientation to the law, its impact on employment, and implementation of those laws are required to demonstrate compliance with the law. Ignorance is no excuse – courts expect that all employers know the law.

Consequences for noncompliance with a law have serious repercussions for both the medical practice and the supervisor. Supervisor prejudice, employer bias, and ignorance can be costly for the medical practice and do not make good business sense. An educational program for new supervisors and an ongoing educational program for current supervisors will help ensure that everyone is current and up to date on correct employment practices.

Appropriate vs. Inappropriate Actions

Some common practices that can be inappropriate in terms of employment revolve around candidate interviews. Knowing the right (and wrong) kinds of questions to ask may seem simple, but in reality, it is quite complex. Questions about the candidate's age, marital status, and place of residence are appropriate for a health physical (which many physicians perform each day), but not for an employment interview. The medical practice executive can help supervisors know how to interview as well as learn what is considered an appropriate action vs. an inappropriate one.

Supervisory Responsibilities

A supervisor is responsible for following the law. Well-meaning intentions to "help out" an older worker by giving higher-paid work to a younger worker because the older worker might be tired, or not promoting a pregnant worker because she needs her rest while pregnant, will lead to employee grievances for discriminatory practices. If a supervisor is ever unsure of the correct practice, he or she should consult with the medical practice executive, who should be conversant with such laws.

Supervisory Review and Monitoring Functions

Management by expectation is a first start toward compliance, but management by inspection provides a practical way to demonstrate compliance with the law. Observing appropriate HR practices helps the medical practice executive know whether a practice is being followed and the areas for which additional education and training may be needed.

Measuring compliance with the law is another way to determine that all HR functions are being followed. Auditing personnel records for I-9 forms and completed employment applications, and reviewing whether all employees have received and signed receipt of the employee handbook are all important measures that the medical practice executive can conduct.

Documentation

Memory does not constitute documentation, nor does the statement, "I'm too busy. I don't have time to document." Documentation is the cornerstone of HR management and the medical practice executive's responsibility, and is a critical element for any follow-up needed on resolving any issue.

Investigation

Sometimes, the medical practice executive needs to conduct an investigation to learn further information before a final decision is made. For example, an employee may have completed the employment application by answering "No" to the question about "Have you ever been convicted of a felony?" However, a background check may reveal that the employee has a record with a conviction. The practice executive needs to investigate the accuracy of the data collected and interview the employee for further information prior to making a decision on any new data. Employee discipline and termination is another supervising function that cannot be overlooked. For further discussion on these skills, see Chapter 2. It is usually the policy of a medical practice to terminate an employee who has falsified information on an employment application.

Maintaining compliance with employment laws is accomplished through continuous review and monitoring of HR policies, procedures, and practices. By keeping current on practices that impact the medical group, the medical practice executive can align organizational needs with HR law. Attention to detail and commitment to compliance become part of the management culture and enable the medical group to function appropriately within the confines of the law.

Chapter 7

Enhancing Knowledge, Skills, and Abilities in Health Care Administration

■ Changing Information Requirements

One of the many facets that make medical practice management both challenging and rewarding is the incredible rate of change in the medico-economics field. New drugs and therapies, new surgical procedures, and new regulatory reforms are announced every day. All of the new drugs and procedures need to be factored into the microeconomic side of the health care equation, and the regulatory changes that affect practices at all levels, from how one recruits new physician partners down to how the medical record clerk angles his or her computer screen. From the practice executive's perspective, these changes present both a challenge and an opportunity. There is no central oversight of medical practice, no universal implementers of new policies or procedures. Accordingly, it is up to the practice executive to keep abreast of all these changes, so that he or she can incorporate change into the practices in ways that are economical, affordable, and compliant with any new laws and regulations.

◼ Change Management Through Continuing Education

Medical practice executives not only need to implement a specific solution to each new change, but, equally important, they need to establish context for change. Often, staff – and even partners – are so absorbed in their own functions that they are not aware of larger trends in the health care or business environment. The practice executive must continue to monitor trends and stay up to date in order to establish context when asking staff or partners to make changes. Knowing there is a Medicare prescription drug benefit, and knowing both how the benefit works and how it is paid for, can help the executive communicate with partners and staff regarding prescribing patterns. Understanding the Internal Revenue Service intermediate sanctions rules can help an executive in the nonprofit sector clarify why additional documentation and scrutiny of business-related expenses are necessary. Understanding the status of class-action lawsuits against hospitals regarding billing practices for the uninsured helps the executive explain why inquiries are being made regarding the group's practices around billing the uninsured.

Executives can keep up with information and change in many ways. The primary methods involve memberships and continuing education. Memberships in such groups as the Medical Group Management Association (MGMA), the American College of Medical Practice Executives (ACMPE), and the Healthcare Financial Management Association (HFMA) provide material such as monthly journals and electronic discussion groups, many tailored to specific needs. In addition, MGMA offers its members access to an online Knowledge Center (mgma.com), a Web portal providing access to literature databases, an article archive, and other information, as well as information products on specific topics, which can be ordered as needed. Every specialty publishes a variety of journals that offer articles and advice regarding practice management issues. In addition, a plethora of nonspecialty-specific journals are aimed at assisting the medical practice with its business, on issues ranging from coding alerts to medical economics. In many cases, monitoring the general press and business press (the daily newspaper, the *Wall Street Journal,* Business Week, and Newsweek, to name a few) can give an executive tips on upcoming knowledge needs, issues, and trends. Most professional organizations also sponsor numerous continuing-education events at which executives can attend various workshops and lectures on subjects they need to learn. These events also offer opportunities to meet with others facing the same or similar challenges and to learn from colleagues how to approach specific issues. In fact, ACMPE even requires its members to document 50 hours of continuing education over a three-year period to maintain certification.

Credentialing and Leadership

Board certification of the medical practice executive acts as a demonstration of the executive's commitment to professionalism, and one of the common principles in all the definitions of professionalism is the necessity to participate in continuing education. By participating in continuing education, the executive makes a statement to the practice's partners, to colleagues, and to staff that the executive values the process of participating in continuing education and is thus of more value, with a higher skill set, than one who does not. As noted earlier, medical practice takes place in a highly credentialed environment, and by holding board certification, the executive demonstrates to the partners and staff a commitment to all of the values of professionalism, including the value of continuing education.

With physicians trained to deliver highly specialized patient care, partners are dependent on the medical practice executive to arrange the business affairs of the practice to achieve the group's goals. Colleagues, both internal and external to the practice, must respect the executive's leadership skills for the practice to thrive. The old adage about the leader without followers is true: If people are unwilling to follow, leaders are unable to lead. Much of the willingness to follow is based on the trust placed in the executive's leadership. Followers, whether they be partners, colleagues, or staff, need to trust a leader's (the practice executive's) skills in order to fully participate in processes.

There are as many different leadership styles as there are leaders, but at some level, leaders have earned the trust of their followers through experience, respect, and special knowledge and skills. In a special 2004 *Business Week* report, "The Future of Work," those careers expected to survive and thrive in the future economy were those positions that required "flexibility, creativity and a commitment to life-long learning."[45] In contrast, positions with regularly recurring, routine work demands were expected to wither away. As cited by author Peter Coy in the *Business Week* report, in "The New Division of Labor: How Computers Are Creating the Next Job Market," Frank Levy of the Massachusetts Institute of Technology and Richard J. Murnane of Harvard state that two kinds of jobs will remain in high demand. The first involves complex pattern recognition, such as spotting business opportunities or dealing with complex systems. The second category relies on complex communication skills, such as managing people, devising advertising campaigns, or selling big-ticket items.

It is clear that a medical practice executive holds responsibilities similar to both of the types that are expected to thrive. In summary, the article's author, Peter Coy, states, "Are you flexible, creative and good with people? You should do fine in tomorrow's job market."[46] The leadership skills an executive develops and exhibits are often what differentiate the successful practice from those practices "just getting by."

■ Promote Ethical Standards for Individual and Organizational Behavior, and Decision Making

Ethical Standards – The Heart of Professional Responsibility

As noted previously in the discussion about professionalism, one of the common threads in all definitions of professionals is adherence to an ethical standard and a definitive statement that individuals will act with integrity. Indeed, some definitions state that the members of a profession will act as ethical enforcement for the rest of the profession. Thus, attorneys have membership in their state bar associations as a prerequisite to licensure, and launch inquiries and investigations through the bar association when one member accuses another of acting unethically. Ethical standards require adherence to a higher standard of action than simple, expedient, and technically correct business actions. Ethical behavior requires adherence to duty and vigilance of action. Ethical behavior means actions are not only legal, but "right" from a variety of perspectives. In some cases, ethical behavior may actually increase the costs of doing business, not only from a vigilance perspective, but because actions are taken that would not be taken absent an ethical standard. In putting patients' interests above those of the practice, in some cases the practice may come out worse off economically. In treating staff fairly, as opposed to simply "what can be gotten away with," a practice sometimes will raise its costs. Investing in quality assurance programs because it is the right thing to do for patients can increase a practice's costs. Nevertheless, doing the right thing is a cost of doing business and is one that the professionally responsible medical practice executive recognizes.

Medical practices sometimes have competing goals, and if not held to high standards, those so-called "structural" conflicts can create opportunities for unethical behavior. Maximizing the partners' incomes can compete with goals of serving the community or treating the staff fairly, and it is up to the executive to uphold that higher standard and recognize and manage the potential conflicts of interest. The professional executive's sense of duty – to patients, to the partners, to the staff, and to the community – is sometimes the last line of defense in guarding against unethical outcomes. Recently in Vermont, a hospital's chief executive officer was sentenced to two years in federal prison for lying to state regulators about the costs of a building expansion. By following his perceived *sole* duty to his employer to get state approval for the project at all costs, he violated ethical principles and even the law. Three others from that hospital's executive team also face criminal charges in that case.[47]

These types of cases illustrate that maintaining ethical standards is a matter of individual integrity and that only by being bound by a sense of professional responsibility and what is right or wrong will an executive truly rise to the level of a professional.

Engage in Professional Networking

Tapping into Networks

Given the complexity of the health care environment, the rapid pace of change, and the increasing specialization of the field, the medical practice executive's ability to tap into an informed network of colleagues and organizations is essential. Whether for physicians, allied health professionals, or medical practice leadership, professional organizations exist at all levels – local, regional, national, and even international. Professional organizations do not have to be limited, however, to the health care environment. Groups at the local level, such as Toastmasters, Jaycees, Rotary, and Lions Clubs, offer an excellent opportunity to network and participate in the business community at large. MGMA and ACMPE, along with their specialty societies and assemblies, offer opportunities at the state and national levels. Among other health care organizations are the HFMA, the American College of Healthcare Executives, and specialty society organizations such as the American College of Cardiology and the American College of Obstetricians and Gynecologists.

Many an executive's reach has been measured by the power of his or her Rolodex or personal digital assistant (PDA) – objects that represent the ability to reach the right person, at the right place, at the right time. With PDAs so ubiquitous in today's business world, the term "Rolodex" might seem archaic, conjuring up an image of a wheeled directory of names and phone numbers. But the idea of the power and capability to contact someone "in the know" through a quick phone call remains the same.

Certainly the power of the e-mail forum (e.g., electronic mailing list) has revolutionized business connectivity, linking individuals and groups of like interests electronically.[48] On an active electronic discussion list, industry news can be instantly distributed, questions can be asked and answered, and a repository of knowledge can be tapped.

In today's complex environment, then, when appropriately tapped, networks offer a powerful professional aid to the medical practice executive.

◢ Develop Effective Interpersonal Skills

An executive who knows himself or herself will be a more effective leader and will recognize the importance of an interpersonal skill set that values and draws out individual and team contributions. Dispelling any doubt about the importance of honing interpersonal skills, the *Business Week* article mentioned earlier identified the ability to "manage people" as a skill set that would ensure an individual's future employment.[49]

The military has certainly understood the need to manage people as well as the value of teamwork. In his book, *Business Is Combat*, author James D. Murphy applies the lessons of a combat pilot to general business management.[50] Murphy points out that it is teams of people who get a fighter plane off the ground, and he lists techniques to improve teamwork, from clearly articulating a mission to punctuality (starting meetings on time) and exercising respect for colleagues (teammates).

Health care, by its very nature, is team oriented; indeed, multidisciplinary teams deliver patient care. From the building maintenance staff to the operating room surgeon, scores, if not hundreds, of staff are involved in the safe and effective delivery of quality health care. The book *The Physician-Manager Alliance* states that "today … the ethical provider is not a solitary physician but a complex health care organization operating under constraints that daily test their commitment to patients."[51] Team management, then, is a critical element in the medical practice executive's success. Effective leadership is the key to developing strong teams, and strong interpersonal skills serve as a foundation for this leadership.[52] Knowledge of team and interpersonal dynamics assists the executive in providing this leadership.

Conclusion

CREATING AN EFFICIENT and effective human resource function is one of the most important activities in a medical practice. The medical practice has to care for its staff and attract and retain the best employees. The human resource function of managing employees and addressing their needs and wants is a constant challenge. A function that exclusively focuses on the employees without an organizational commitment to increase patient satisfaction through a cultural change, however, will ultimately fall short on improving service.

Human Resource Management must focus its commitment to a service culture that brings physicians and employees together to improve patient, physician, and employee satisfaction. A commitment focused on service to people (patients, employees, and physicians alike) fosters a transformation to service excellence. The medical practice that focuses its effort on excellent service will differentiate itself from the competition. The human resource function can help facilitate the accountability of that service from physicians, administrators, and staff. The shared commitment and cooperation of these groups is critical for a culture of service to evolve meaningfully and to make a difference.

A well-run medical practice with a strong vision, mission, goals, and objectives will use its human resource function to develop, implement, and maintain excellent programs in salary and wage administration, benefits administration, procedures and policies, recruitment, appraisal and evaluation, employee relations, training and development, and reward and recognition. The key to that success will be grounded in excellent service and quality patient care.

Exercises

THESE QUESTIONS have been retired from the ACMPE Essay Exam question bank. Because there are so many ways to handle various situations, there are no "right" answers, and thus, no answer key. Use these questions to help you practice responses in different scenarios.

1. You are the administrator of a group that has historically used registered nurses as its sole clinical support staff. You realize this might not be an ideal staffing model.

   Explain how you would evaluate your staffing mix and how you would implement any subsequent changes.

2. You are the administrator of a primary care practice that
    derives 40 percent of its revenues from capitated contracts.
    The group recently lost several of its physicians to active
    duty when their National Guard unit was activated. The
    group is unsure how to manage the capacity in the interim.

    Describe how you would handle this situation.

3. You are the administrator of a medical practice. A physician-owner has demanded an increase in an employee's salary because he believes the employee is irreplaceable. The employee has indicated that she will leave unless she gets a raise. The supervisor's performance reviews of the employee, however, do not justify the increase.

Describe how you would resolve this situation.

4. You are the new administrator of a medical practice. The group does not have a formal wage administration plan. The physicians have set salaries for their own staff and have created disparate wages among similar positions. A female employee files a formal grievance that a male employee in a similar position with less seniority is being paid more than she is.

   Describe how you would handle this situation.

5. You are the administrator of an oncology group of four
    male and two female physicians. The office has two pods
    of exam rooms shared by male and female physicians. Each
    physician has one nurse to assist daily with the patients.
    One of the nurses left a note on your desk stating that she
    intends to file a sexual harassment complaint against one
    of the oncologists who works in the same pod. The nurse
    states that the physician constantly tells "sexist" and inap-
    propriate jokes to staff and patients.

    What course of action would you take in this situation?

Notes

1. Reprinted from *MGMA Connexion,* October 2007, with permission of Medical Group Management Association. All rights reserved.

2. Reduce Physician Turnover and Improve Your Bottom Line – Physicians Speak up About Retention Issues, 2006, www.locumtenens.com/retention (accessed March 15, 2007).

3. Ibid.

4. Patients, Physicians and Employees: Satisfaction Trifecta Brings Bottom Line Results, Press Ganey, 2005, www.pressganey.com/files/roiv2.pdf (accessed March 3, 2007).

5. Reduce Physician Turnover and Improve Your Bottom Line – Physicians Speak up About Retention Issues, (2006) www.locumtenens.com/retention (accessed March 15, 2007).

6. Adapted from M. Vuletich, "Find Dr. Right, Then Treat Him or Her Right," *MGMA e-Source*, April 2007.

7. This section was written by Susan Wendling-Aloi, MPA, FACMPE, MGMA member, and regional manager of operations, Sonix Diagnostic Imaging, Chatham, N.J., and is reprinted with permission from MGMA, as derived from a professional paper submitted to the American College of Medical Practice Executives in partial fulfillment of requirements to achieve the certification of Fellow.

8. Hansen, http://www2.mgma.com/literature/

9. R. Redling, More Than Salary Necessary to Keep Physicians on Board, 2001 *MGM Update*, 40(6): 1.

10. R. D. Hansen, What Makes a Successful Medical Group? *MGM Update* 2001, 40(15): 6.

11. Ibid.

12. G.S. Benedict, "Chapter 5: Organization and Governance" in *The Development and Management of Medical Groups* (Colorado: Medical Group Management Association and American Medical Association, 1996), 89–90.

13. This section is reprinted from *HR Policies and Procedures Manual for Medical Practices*, 4th edition, copyright 2007, pages 267–289, with permission of Medical Group Management Association. All rights reserved.

14. *Uniform Guidelines on Employee Selection Procedures* (Washington, DC: Bureau of National Affairs, 1979).

15. Lawrence F. Wolper, *Physician Practice Management: Essential Operational and Financial Knowledge* (Sudbury, MA: Jones and Bartlett, 2005), 154, 160–161.

16. U.S. Bureau of Labor Statistics, "Census of Fatal Occupational Injuries (CFOI) – Current and Revised Data," www.bls.gov/iif/oshcfoi1.htm.

17. Stephen L. Wagner, "Defining the ACMPE Fellow," *College View* (Fall 2003): 27–30.

18. U.S. Congressional Budget Office, *How Many People Lack Health Insurance and for How Long?* (Washington, DC: U.S. Congressional Budget Office, Health and Human Resources Division, May 2003).

19. Alicia H. Munnell, Francesca Golub-Sass, and Anthony Webb, "What Moves the National Retirement Risk Index? A Look Back and an Update," *An Issue in Brief: Center for Retirement Research at Boston College*, January 2007, Number 2007-1.

20. Thomas J. Stanley and William D. Danko, *The Millionaire Next Door* (Atlanta: Longstreet Press, 1996), 74–77.

21. Lisa Smith, "The Generation Gap," *Investopedia.com,* July 17, 2006, www.investopedia.com/printable.asp?=articles/pf/06/generationgap.asp (accessed Jan. 20, 2007).

22. U.S. Department of Labor Bureau of Labor Statistics, "Employee Benefits Survey" http://data.bls.gov/cgi/surveymost (accessed Jan. 22, 2007).

23. "Fiduciary Responsibilities," U.S. Department of Labor, www.dol.gov/dol/topic (accessed Jan. 23, 2007).

24. Kevin J. Donovan, "Defined Benefit Plan Design," in *The CPA's Guide to Retirement Plans for Small Businesses,* ed. Gary S. Lesser (New York: American Institute of Certified Public Accountants, 2004), 217–218.

25. Munnell, Golub-Sass, and Webb, 4.

26. Donovan, 217–218.

27. Richard A. Naegele, "Tax Qualified Retirement Plans and Fringe Benefits," in *Physician Practice Management: Essential Operational and Financial Knowledge,* ed. Lawrence F. Wolper (Sudbury, MA: Jones and Bartlett, 2005), 572.

28. Ibid., 570.

29. Lawrence C. Starr, "Internal Revenue Code Section 401(k) and Safe Harbor 401(k) Plan Design," in *The CPA's Guide to Retirement Plans for Small*

Businesses, ed. Gary S. Lesser (New York: American Institute of Certified Public Accountants, 2004), 189–191.

30. Naegele, 573.

31. Ibid., 574–575.

32. Ibid., 572–573.

33. Gary S. Lesser, "ERISA Fiduciary Considerations," in *The CPAs Guide to Retirement Plans for Small Businesses,* ed. Gary S. Lesser (New York: American Institute of Certified Public Accountants, 2004): 474–475.

34. Naegele, 577.

35. Cynthia Van Bogaert, "FYI: Investment Advice for Participants," http://boardmanlawfirm.com/fyi/09_28_06.html (accessed Jan. 22, 2007).

36. Lesser, 476.

37. Naegele, 577.

38. Lesser, 10–11.

39. Ibid., 135–161.

40. Naegele, 570–571.

41. Lesser, 165–167.

42. "Health Plans & Benefits," U.S. Department of Labor, www.dol.gov/dol/topic/ (accessed Jan. 22, 2007).

43. 2005 Instructions for Form 5500 Annual Return/Report of Employee Benefit Plan, Internal Revenue Service, 1.

44. Lesser, 389–93.

45. Peter Coy, "The Future of Work," *Business Week* (Mar.22, 2005): 50.

46. Ibid.

47. Tony Fong, "Strong Message: Fletcher Allen Official Received Two-Year Sentence," *Modern Healthcare* (May 2, 2005): 17.

48. "Glossary of Selected Distance Learning Terms and Phrases," www.trainingfinder.org/DCD_lingo (accessed June 17, 2005).

49. Coy, "The Future of Work," 50.

50. James D. Murphy, *Business Is Combat* (New York: HarperCollins, 2000), 15.

51. Stephen M. Davidson, Marion McCollom, and Janelle Heineke, *The Physician-Manager Alliance* (San Francisco: Jossey-Bass, 1996), 72.

52. Patrick Lencioni, *The FIVE Dysfunctions of a TEAM* (San Francisco: Jossey-Bass, 2002), 195.

Glossary

affirmative action – A set of public policies designed to help eliminate discrimination based on race, color, religion, sex, or national origin.

Americans with Disabilities Act of 1990 (ADA) – A federal civil rights law designed to prevent discrimination and allow people with disabilities to participate fully in all aspects of society.

arbitration – A process by which opposing parties present a dispute to an impartial arbitrator to determine a decision.

Consolidated Omnibus Budget Reconciliation Act of 1985 (COBRA) – A federal employment insurance law that requires employers to provide a time-limited health insurance premium to any employee who leaves the organization.

employee assistance program (EAP) – A benefit offered by employers that provides help to employees to address personal issues that may impact employee performance.

Employee Retirement Income Security Act of 1974 (ERISA) – A federal law that sets minimum standards for voluntary established pension and health plans to protect plan participants.

Family and Medical Leave Act of 1993 (FMLA) – A law requiring covered employers to provide up to 12 weeks of unpaid, job-protected leave to "eligible" employees for certain family and medical reasons.

Federal Insurance Contributions Act (FICA) – A section of the Internal Revenue Code that requires a portion of a worker's paycheck to be deducted to support the Social Security and Medicare programs.

401(k) plan – Voluntary investment plan in which the employer defers employee compensation to a special fund for future use at retirement.

full-time-equivalent (FTE) – A term used to describe the number of hours considered to be the minimum for an employee to work in a normal work week; this can be 37.5, 40, or 50 hours per week, or some other standard.

Gainsharing – A reward system for increased productivity by which employee pay increases are based on organizational productivity or cost reductions.

Health Insurance Portability and Accountability Act of 1996 (HIPAA) – Health care legislation that mandates the safety, security, and protection of patient data, specifically addressing storage, dissemination, and access to protected health information.

Internal Revenue Service (IRS) – An agency of the federal government that taxes people and organizations for services.

IRS Code Section 457 – Nonqualified, deferred compensation plans established by state and local government and tax-exempt employers.

job task – A high-level function describing a key component of a position.

mediation – A formal process in which a professional mediator works with two parties and seeks to achieve agreement.

National Labor Relations Act of 1935 (NLRA) – Legislation passed to protect employees' rights to unionize. The National Labor Relations Board was created to implement and enforce the NLRA.

Occupational Safety and Health Act of 1970 – Legislation that established the nationwide, federal Occupational Safety and Health Administration program to protect the work force from job-related death, injury, and illness.

pay grades/steps – Parts of a compensation system. A "grade" is assigned to a specific position based on the required skills, qualifications, and requirements needed for job performance. These grades are placed into progressive "steps."

profit sharing – A compensation system by which the employees of a medical practice receive a predetermined share of the organization's profits.

severance pay – A predetermined amount of money, usually based on length of service within an organization, that an employee may receive if his or her position is terminated.

strategic plan – A written document, usually created for a three- to five-year period, that communicates the medical practice's vision for the future.

workers' compensation – A state-mandated form of insurance covering workers injured in job-related accidents. In some states, the state is the insurer; in other states, insurance must be acquired from commercial insurance firms. Insurance rates are based on a number of factors, including salaries, firm history, and risk of occupation.

Index

Note: (ex.) indicates exhibit.